The Activity Year Book

of related interest

How to Make Your Care Home Fun
Simple Activities for People of All Abilities
Kenneth Agar
ISBN 978 1 84310 952 5

Understanding Care Homes
A Research and Development Perspective
Sue Davies, Katherine Froggatt and Julienne Meyer
ISBN 978 1 84310 553 4

Involving Families in Care Homes
A Relationship-Centred Approach to Dementia Care
Bob Woods, John Keady and Diane Seddon
ISBN 978 1 84310 229 8
Bradford Dementia Group Good Practice Guides

Design for Nature in Dementia Care
Garuth Chalfont
ISBN 978 1 84310 571 8
Bradford Dementia Group Good Practice Guides

The Pool Activity Level (PAL) Instrument for Occupational Profiling
A Practical Resource for Carers of People with Cognitive Impairment
3rd edition
Jackie Pool
ISBN 978 1 84310 594 7
Bradford Dementia Group Good Practice Guides

Remembering Yesterday, Caring Today
Reminiscence in Dementia Care: A Guide to Good Practice
Pam Schweitzer and Errollyn Bruce
Foreword by Faith Gibson
ISBN 978 1 84310 649 4
Bradford Dementia Group Good Practice Guides

The Activity Year Book

A Week by Week Guide for Use in Elderly Day and Residential Care

ANNI BOWDEN AND NANCY LEWTHWAITE

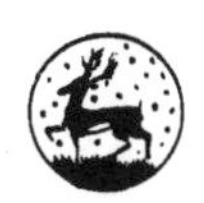

Jessica Kingsley Publishers
London and Philadelphia

First published in 2009
by Jessica Kingsley Publishers
116 Pentonville Road
London N1 9JB, UK
and
400 Market Street, Suite 400
Philadelphia, PA 19106, USA

www.jkp.com

Library of Congress Cataloging in Publication Data

Bowden, Anni.
The activity year book : a week by week guide for use in elderly day and residential care / Anni Bowden and Nancy Lewthwaite.
p. cm.
ISBN 978-1-84310-963-1 (pb : alk. paper)
1. Older people--Care. 2. Older people--Recreation. 3. Older people--Services for. 4. Older people--Institutional care. I. Lewthwaite, Nancy. II. Title.
RA999.R42B69 2009
613'.0438--dc22

2008029312

British Library Cataloguing in Publication Data
A CIP catalogue record for this book is available from the British Library

ISBN 978 1 84310 963 1

Printed and bound in Great Britain by
Printwise (Haverhill) Ltd, Suffolk

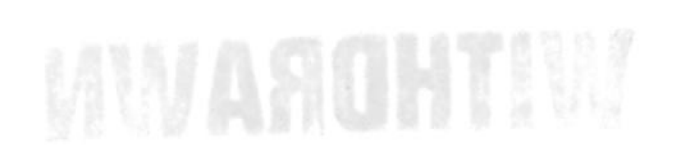

Contents

Acknowledgements

We would like to thank Carolyn Swan, Judith Queenborough, Valerie Eaton Griffith, Elizabeth Pepys, Sue Miller and Puzzler Media for their generosity in allowing us to use their wonderful material, but most of all we wish to thank all those wonderful older folk we have met in our working life, who have inspired and humbled us with their true grit and sense of humour.

Getting Started

We all know that people who are engaged in some kind of activity, who are occupied, have a happier and more fulfilled life, but we don't always know how to go about providing the right type of activity for them. This book can help to give you ideas and ways of doing just that. Some may be more useful than others, but you can adapt most to your own circumstances. The majority of the ideas cost little more than your time and can be as easy as simply replanning your day – but all of them are diverting and (we think) mostly *fun*!

How to run a group

The right group leader is most important

A designated activity organiser is essential as the person who will prepare and evaluate the activities. Time should be allowed for this, possibly Friday afternoon, ready for the next week. He or she should feel confident in presenting to a number of people, have an outgoing personality and be able to support both colleagues and group members. Our own activity organiser reached the point of being unable to go anywhere without wondering how what she saw or did could be used in a group activity!

The group

Do invite people to the group – some people hate to be a 'joiner' but may still decide to come in next time when they hear the laughter!

A circle is the best way of ensuring that everyone can see the presenter and the flipchart. Speak clearly and slowly to make sure everyone hears and understands the activities. Allow plenty of time for people to answer questions and complete the activities.

Staffing the group

At least two staff members are needed to run a group, in case someone requires the toilet, needs help to read or write, has hearing difficulties (a microphone can be really useful if many people are hearing impaired), or needs things explaining more. Prepare the circle of chairs before the group begins. It is best if staff sit opposite each other in the circle. It is important that everything is to hand before running the group, and that facilitators know what they are doing.

When making copies of items, enlarging them may make them more user-friendly.

One staff member will be the 'scribe' and write on the flipchart – so it is essential that they feel comfortable in writing and spelling. We found it useful to have a stack of magazines for group members to 'rest' paper on for writing.

All the items required for any activity should be prepared in advance and ready to use. Maybe a special group box will help to achieve this.

When leading the reminiscence and discussion, let people have their say, as they like to share life experiences. Encourage the group to listen and ask questions. Sometimes it may be necessary to use the prompts or your own/family experiences to get the group to relax about the topic.

We found we really appreciated the group more as individuals when we learnt of the hardships they had overcome. We also found some amazing hidden talents and skills. This helped us to make fewer snap judgements of people and reduced unconscious ageism – which in turn led to everyone becoming much closer.

It is essential that time is given for the group members to answer. Give support to enable them to do so, and also encourage group members to allow each other time and support. We found this very soon happened spontaneously and really created group bonding. It is important that the group and *not* the staff answer the questions! If either the questions or the answers provoke discussion, let this develop as a natural spin-off to the group's enjoyment.

All staff must respect the importance of the group and should only interrupt an activity if it is absolutely necessary. They should also make sure that any noisy work or discussion takes place away from the group room.

Each group session follows a similar pattern:

1. outline of the theme for the week
2. reminiscence and discussion
3. opportunity to share information
4. linked quizzes, word games
5. observation activity or a poem.

For people with memory problems or dementia there are activities that have a sensory component, or more physical games such as adapted 'beetle' or 'target' games.

Each of the following weekly guides begins with a list of equipment required.

The activities

Aims of the activities

- socialising and interacting with others
- communication skills practice – listening, taking turns and speaking

- sharing experience and reminiscence
- use of both short- and long-term memory
- physical activity and hand–eye coordination
- use of cognitive skills
- *fun* – for staff too! – remember, laughter has been proved to be the best medicine.

Evaluating the activities

It is a good idea to spend a few minutes after the group to discuss how it went, what worked, what didn't, what can you make easier, more fun? There is an evaluation sheet at the back of the book, which may be useful. We entered group attendance and reactions in clients' notes – this can be very positive for letting relatives know that their loved ones are happy – especially if the client forgets to tell them what they have been doing during the week. It may also be useful for NVQ. It will underline the importance of activities to all staff, and increase a client-centred approach.

In a residential setting it would be possible to use all the activities by using just the reminiscence and discussion on Day 1, then introducing one activity, with a reminder of the theme, each day for the rest of the week. People are more easily tired and lose concentration more easily when they are frail.

In day care, if people attend more than one day per week they can easily join in the reminiscence session by listening to others, which may stimulate more memories for themselves, and they can join in any activities that were not used on their previous attendance. (It is not necessary to complete the whole programme each day, far better to let things flow naturally, if something is going well, and save unused activities for another day.) The book is in monthly segments, but it is not necessary to follow this rigidly. However, it may be useful until the activity organiser has grown in confidence and begins to 'pick and mix' or invent their own themed weeks.

The following books were used in planning the activities:

- *The Stroke Activity Book* compiled by Valerie Eaton Griffith, Elizabeth Pepys and Sue Miller (1992). Published by the Stroke Association. (Now unfortunately out of print.)
- *Language and Word Activities* by Judith Queenborough (1998). Published by Speechmark Publishing, Bicester.
- *Mental Aerobics* by Nancy J. Lewthwaite. Published by Nancy in 1986.
- *More Mental Aerobics* by Nancy J. Lewthwaite. Also published by Nancy in 1993. (Nancy can be contacted via her website www.mentalaerobics.net)
- *Puzzler Magazine* Puzzler Media Ltd, Redhill.

Some other useful books:

Remembering Yesterday, Caring Today (2008) by Pam Schweitzer and Errollyn Bruce. Published by Jessica Kingsley Publishers, London.

The Pool (PAL) Instrument for Occupational Profiling Activity Level (2007) by Jackie Pool Published by Jessica Kingsley Publishers, London.

The active day

1. Meet and greet – welcome each person by name (first name if permission has been given). This is a really positive approach, as often people who live alone will not have heard their own name spoken for some time, and this will serve to affirm their individuality and sense of self.
2. Over coffee ask each person how they are today, have an exchange of news – theirs and yours – and discuss any important news of the day. Encourage conversation between clients.
3. Bingo…to accommodate all those people who enjoy this game – there are quite a number!
4. Walk into dining room for lunch.
5. Walk back into lounge area for snooze, magazine/newspaper reading, lunchtime TV, tabletop games such as Scrabble, whist, draughts.
6. Armchair exercises – to get the circulation going.
7. Cup of tea.
8. Themed activity session for an hour.
9. Walk into dining room for tea.

Walking from one area to another can dramatically increase exercise levels for the day, involving balance practice and getting in and out of chairs, as well as mobilising.

Activities for January

Week 1 – Twelfth Night

Equipment: flipchart, pens, paper, three wastebins marked gold, frankincense and myrrh, three beanbags, copies of 'The carol singers' (page 17).

1. Reminiscence and discussion

Ask the group what they used to do at this time of year, can they remember any of the customs about the taking down of Christmas decorations? Was it bad luck to keep them up longer than Twelfth Night? What happened if they didn't? (In some places the decorations had to remain until Easter to counteract the bad luck. Was it the same for them?) Twelfth Night – 6 January – was traditionally known as the last day of Christmas festivities, and the decorations – usually a tree – would be taken down at midnight on 5 January and burnt, followed by singing, eating and drinking until dawn. A 'surprise' cake would be baked, with a bean hidden inside, and whoever found it would be crowned King or Queen of the Revels. It is said that on that day the Three Wise Men reached Bethlehem and gave their gifts to Jesus. Can the group name the Three Wise Men? (Melchior, Balthazar, Caspar.) What gifts did they bring? (Gold, frankincense and myrrh.) Can the group think of any carols associated with this time? ('As with gladness men of old', 'We three kings of Orient are'.) Do they remember the irreverent version they sang at school? 'We three kings of Orient are, One on a motor bike, one in a car, One on a scooter blowing his hooter, Following yonder star.')

In the Christian calendar Twelfth Night is known as the Feast of Epiphany, and early Christians believed Jesus was baptised on this day. This makes it a popular day for christenings. Any in the group or their families baptised on this day? Royal epiphany gifts are distributed every year at a ceremony dating from medieval times in the Chapel Royal at St James Palace on 6 January. Two Gentlemen Ushers offer, on behalf of the Queen, gifts of gold, frankincense and myrrh in silk bags placed on an alms dish. The gold is now given in the form of 25 gold sovereigns, which are exchanged for £25 in cash to be distributed to the aged poor.

Plough Monday is the first Monday after 6 January and was called thus because it was the day farm work was resumed after the Twelve Days of Christmas and spring ploughing began. This is a rhyme that was said by country folk at this time:

'Plough Monday, next after the Twelfth tide is past
Bids out with the plough, the worst husband is last.'

Plough Tide was one of the Church's agricultural services during the year, and on Plough Sunday services are held in rural areas when the plough is brought into the Church and blessed and prayers for a bountiful harvest are said.

Weather signs were carefully noted, as it was believed they would be an indication of the weather for the rest of the year. Cold weather was wished for, as the old proverb said 'If January six be summerly gay, 'twill be winterly weather till beginning of May.'

2. Proverbs and sayings quiz

Ask the group members in turn to complete the following:

1. A penny for your...thoughts.
2. Too many cooks...spoil the broth.
3. Two's company...three's a crowd.
4. There's no smoke...without fire.
5. First come...first served.
6. Easy come...easy go.
7. The early bird...catches the worm.
8. A rolling stone...gathers no moss.
9. It never rains...but what it pours.
10. Honesty is...the best policy.
11. It's no use...crying over spilt milk.
12. All's well...that ends well.
13. Absence makes...the heart grow fonder.
14. Let sleeping dogs...lie.
15. Early to bed...early to rise makes a man healthy, wealthy and wise.
16. A poor workman...blames his tools.
17. Every cloud...has a silver lining.
18. Mighty oaks...from little acorns grow.
19. You can't teach an old dog...new tricks.
20. Curiosity...killed the cat.
21. You don't put new wine...in old bottles.
22. Marry in haste...repent at leisure.
23. The course of true love...never runs smooth.

24. United we stand...divided we fall.
25. A friend in need...is a friend indeed.
26. Penny wise...pound foolish.
27. You can take a horse to water...but you can't make him drink.
28. Enough is as good...as a feast.
29. While the cat's away...the mice will play.
30. Children should be seen...and not heard.
31. A stitch in time...saves nine.
32. Fools rush in...where angels fear to tread.
33. People in glass houses...shouldn't throw stones.
34. Empty vessels...make the most noise.
35. A bird in the hand...is worth two in the bush.
36. Red sky at night...shepherd's delight.
37. Red sky in the morning...sailor's warning.
38. He who laughs last...laughs longest.
39. Jack of all trades...master of none.
40. More haste...less speed.
41. All that glitters...is not gold.
42. An apple a day...keeps the doctor away.
43. In for a penny...in for a pound.
44. Still waters...run deep.
45. Where there's life...there's hope.
46. Time...and tide wait for no man.
47. Pride...goes before a fall.
48. To err...is human.
49. To forgive...is divine.
50. One swallow...does not a summer make.
51. Cast not a clout...till May is out (this is the May blossom not the month of May).
52. You can't paint...black white.
53. A change...is as good as a rest.
54. You can't make a silk...purse from a sow's ear.
55. Necessity...is the mother of invention.
56. Robbing...Peter to pay Paul.
57. Don't cast your pearls...before swine.

Add more from staff/group.

3. Predictions for the New Year

Give each member of the group a paper and pen and ask them to write down any predictions they feel they could make for the coming year. Collect and read them to the group and keep them in a safe place to be referred to if they come to fruition. Using the flipchart, ask the group for their wishes to change the world for the better.

4. Three Kings target game

In three teams named after the Three Kings, each person in turn has three throws with a beanbag at each bin. They have to get *frankincense* and *myrrh* before going for *gold*. The team taking the fewest throws are Kings of the Revels for the day.

5. Spot the differences: The carol singers

Give everyone a copy of the quiz on page 17.

6. See how many words can be made from: TWELFTH NIGHT.

Week 2 – Winter

Equipment: flipchart, pens, paper, 'feely bag' (with contents), sponge balls covered in cottonwool, plastic bottles.

1. Reminiscence and discussion

Talk with the group about the winters they have experienced. Can they recall the really bad winters we used to have? What happened to them during the bad weather? How did they cope? What form of heating did they have? (NB this is a good time to check that everyone has received their heating allowance and whether they are all keeping their homes warm enough and dressing warmly. Also an opportunity to discuss the dangers of hypothermia and hand out leaflets.)

How did they prevent their pipes freezing? Did anyone get 'Jack Frost' pictures on the inside of their bedroom windows? Was there any heating in the bedroom? Do they still sleep with no heating and the window open? How did they warm the beds? Electric blanket? Hot-water bottle? Anyone have a stone hot-water bottle? Did they have special warm clothing? Was it like the specialist insulated clothing available now or just extra layers? What games did they play in the snow? How did they make a snowman? Did they have snowball fights? Can anyone ski? Has anyone been on a skiing holiday? Did they have sledges? Were they homemade? Can anyone ice-skate? Did the ponds and lakes freeze well enough to allow this? What kind of food kept them warm? (Porridge, rice pudding, steam puddings, stew and

Answers: In right-hand picture – girl's shoes are white, ribbons missing from end and top of plaits, father's hand missing, collar missing, hair is white and teeth different; dog has lost tail and teeth and his nose is white; mother has lost part of her hair, necklace and bottom of cardigan; little boy has no buttons and his shoes are white.

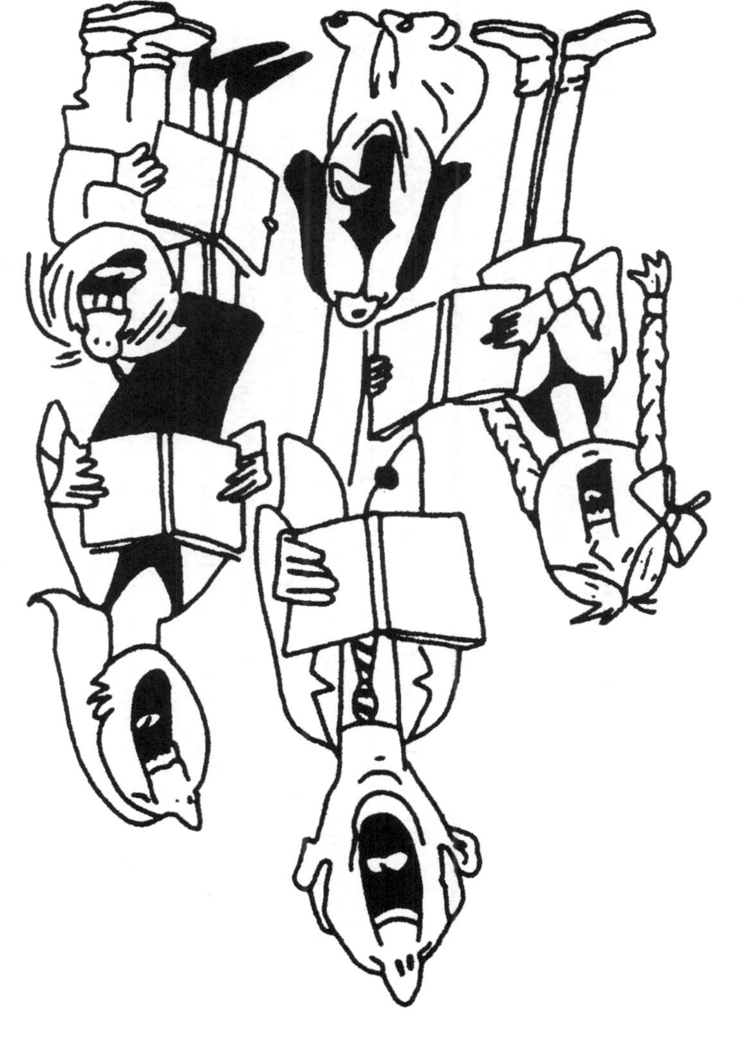

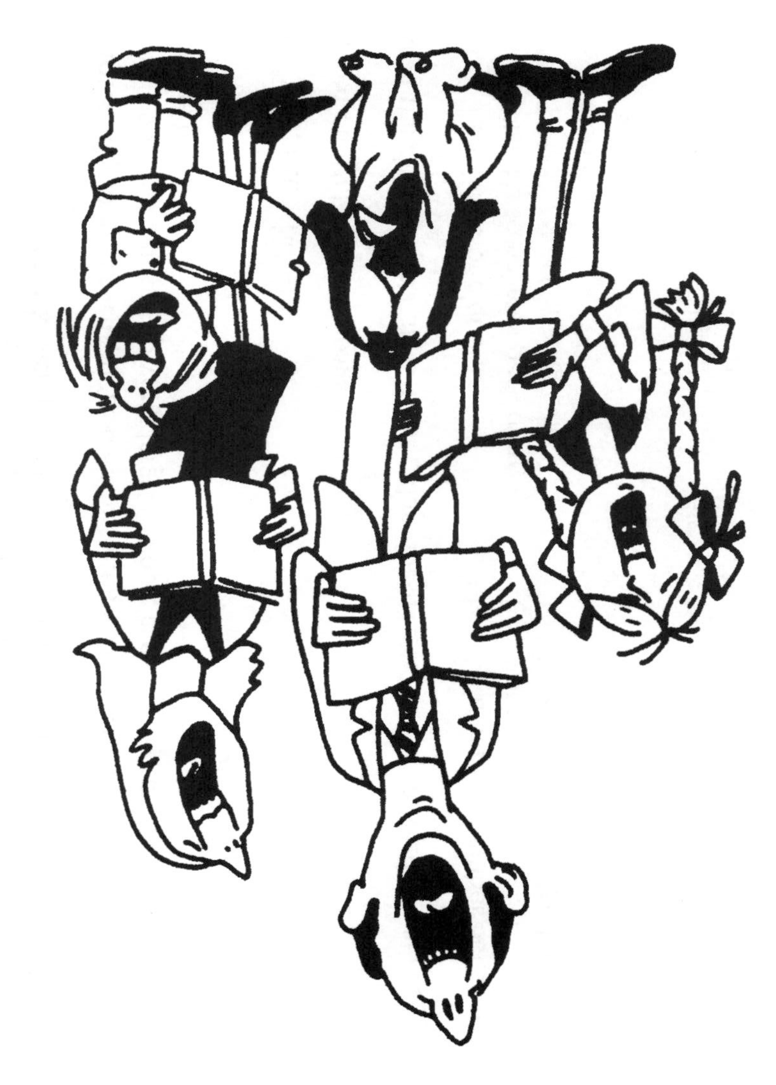

dumplings.) Do they still like this kind of 'comfort' food even today in the winter? Ask what everyone had for breakfast today.

How did they travel to school in the winters? What do they think about how transport deals with the bad weather? Has anyone ever had a bad skid in the snow? How did they cope with it? Are people afraid of walking in the bad conditions? Warn people of the risks of clearing snow. (There is an increase in heart attacks after a snowfall because of path clearing.) They should also be very careful walking on icy paths.

Did people suffer coughs and colds in the winter? What home remedies did they use? Do people feel the climate is changing? As some evidence of this, in the late 1800s and early 1900s fairs were held on frozen lakes and rivers. Do they believe we are suffering from climate change? Any suggestions on possible cause and what we can all do to help.

2. A storm of winter words

On flipchart, with the group responding in turn, record all the words they can think of that remind them of winter. At the day centre a running total can be kept for the week to give a target to beat.

3. Wintertime feely bag and snowball game

Divide the group into two and then take it turn to do the two activities.

Feely bag – in a plastic bag place a hot-water bottle stopper, glove, candle, matchbox, piece of coal, woolly hat, scarf, pine cone, piece of fur, plus any other wintery items. Pass the bag round the group and ask each person to select an item by touch.

Snowball game – cover sponge balls in cottonwool to resemble snowballs, arrange empty plastic bottles as ten-pin bowling targets. People can either sit in chairs or stand to throw or roll the balls.

4. Winter 'What am I?'

(based on *Mental Aerobics* page 265)

Read the clues one at a time. If the group doesn't get the answer read the next clue.

1. I am made of glass.
   Blue tits sometimes peck at my top.
   I used to stand on everyone's doorstep.
   milk bottle

11. I am made of rubber but sometimes stone.
    I am filled with water that is hot.
    I keep your bed warm.
    hot-water bottle

2. I can be made of wood or plastic.
I am best down hills.
I work best on snow.
sledge

3. I am woolly.
I often have a pompom.
I keep your ears warm.
winter hat

4. I am sharp and slippery.
I am metal.
I waltz well.
skates

5. I am chocolate.
I am warm.
I am lovely at bedtime!
cocoa

6. I crackle and sometimes spit.
I can make toast.
I am warm but need feeding.
fire

7. I am full of holes.
I am toasted.
I taste better with butter but some have jam or honey on me.
crumpet

8. I am made of wine and brandy.
I have cloves and cinnamon added.
I am served warm.
mulled wine

9. I have a carrot and coal.
I wear a scarf and have a pipe.
I am white and cold.
snowman

10. People stand on me.
I am long and come in pairs.
I go very fast on snow.
skis

12. I am green and prickly.
I have small red berries.
I deck the halls.
holly

13. I am worn on hands.
I don't have fingers.
I am welcome in winter.
mittens

14. I am named after a general.
I am made of rubber.
I am worn on the feet.
Wellington boots

15. I am from the citrus family.
I am in season in wintertime
I am smaller than an orange.
clementine/satsuma

16. I have a hard exterior.
My inside looks like a brain.
I am a hard one to crack.
walnut

17. I have six sides.
I am made of ice.
We are all different.
snowflake

18. I belong to a pair.
You put me on at night.
I keep your feet nice and warm.
bed socks

19. I keep your food fresh.
I am usually white.
You find me in the kitchen.
fridge

20. I am associated with bees.
Wee Willy Winky had one.
I am handy in a power cut.
candle

Add more of your own.

5. Winter fun quiz

(based on *Mental Aerobics* page 320)

1. Water drops frozen into crystals…snow
2. The shortest day…21 December
3. A large white animal of the frozen North…polar bear
4. When it is very cold this appears around the moon…halo
5. What many birds do to avoid winter…migrate
6. A dessert that is cold in the middle but baked in the oven…baked Alaska
7. The winter home of the Inuit…igloo
8. The coldest part of the world…Antarctica
9. A fierce storm in winter is a…blizzard
10. No two are ever alike…snowflake
11. Frosty is a…snowman (can the group sing his song?)
12. This machine clears the roads…snowplough
13. Another word for a sledge…toboggan
14. What snow does in the wind…drifts
15. Frosty weather is sometimes described as there being a – in the air…nip
16. A mixture of rain and snow…sleet
17. Zero visibility in snow…a whiteout
18. Freezing temperature…0° Centigrade or 32° Fahrenheit
19. The breed of rescue dog used in the Alps…St Bernard
20. Another name for the aurora borealis…the northern lights

6. A winter mix

Write these anagrams one at a time on the flipchart. The group has pen and paper to write down their answers.

CEI	ice	HEITABNER	hibernate
KGNIIS	skiing	TOH RWEAT LEBOTT	hot-water bottle
STORF	frost	HCOGU	cough
WSNO	snow	SGELVO	gloves
ULF	flu	FSCRA	scarf
ZDRAZILB	blizzard	DCLO	cold
TNOAGGBO SREID	toboggan rides	BLLAWSON	snowball
MSANNOW	snowman	CEI YHEOCK	ice hockey

PPERYILS	slippery	TSOFRTIEB	frostbite
YWHEIKS	whisky	CCLESII	icicles

Add more of your own.

7. Winter poem

Ask the group if they would like to write a poem on wintertime, read the following poem as inspiration; then, with permission, read theirs. They may even be good enough to publish in local papers or magazines, etc.

Stopping by Woods on a Snowy Evening
Whose woods these are I think I know
His house is in the village though,
He will not see me stopping here
To watch his woods fill up with snow.

My little horse must think it queer
To stop without a farmhouse near
Between the woods and frozen lake
The darkest evening of the year.

He gives his harness bells a shake
To ask if there is some mistake.
The only other sound's the sweep
Of easy wind and downy flake.

The woods are lovely. Dark and deep,
But I have promises to keep,
And miles to go before I sleep,
And miles to go before I sleep.

Robert Frost

8. See how many words can be made from: TOBOGGAN RIDES.

Week 3 – Burns' night

(or exchange activities with last week in November for St Andrew's Day)

Equipment: flipchart, paper, pens, 'tastes of Scotland' – shortbread, haggis, neeps (turnips) and tatties (mashed potatoes), porridge, Irn Bru, whisky (to sniff), oatmeal biscuits, Dundee cake, Edinburgh rock, drop scones (in a care home setting, or if people come to the centre more than once, it may be an idea to offer one or two Scottish delicacies each day), CD of Scottish music, poems of Robbie Burns.

1. Reminiscence and discussion

Using the flipchart to record responses, ask everyone what they think when they think of Scotland. (In case there is difficulty, here are some prompts: clans, bagpipes, tartan, haggis, Gaelic, Bonnie Prince Charlie, Loch Ness Monster, burn, heather, Edinburgh Tattoo, tam-o'-shanter, Hebrides, dirk, caber tossing, sporran, Robert the Bruce and the spider, whisky, Roamin' in the Gloamin', Harris Tweed, crofters, John o' Groats, fishing, Billy Connolly.)

How many people have been to Scotland for a holiday – how did they travel? Were there midges? Rain? What did they think about the scenery? Where did they stay? Hotel, B&B, tent, caravan, friends or family?

How do the English sometimes describe the Scots? Has the group found this alleged meanness true? Can anyone in the group recall the money-saving tips they used when their children were small and money was tight? Any hints on how to manage on a pension?

THE PATRON SAINT OF SCOTLAND

St Andrew was one of the twelve disciples and was a fisherman, along with his brother Peter. After the crucifixion of Christ he went to Greece to preach Christianity, and here he was crucified for his faith on a cross shaped like an X. The cross on the Scottish flag commemorates this.

In the early days of Christianity people collected relics of saints, such as their bones or articles associated with them, to help them honour and worship the holy men and women. A man was carrying the bones of St Andrew to Scotland when his ship was wrecked on the Fife coast, and the spot where the ship foundered became the town of St Andrews. A cathedral was built there, starting in 1160 and taking 158 years to complete. Another legend says that two monks from the North of England went to Rome for the relics and passed them to the king of Scotland (who was Angus McFergus) in 731 AD.

The Scottish flag is called 'the Saltaire' and the white cross is used because St Andrew appeared in a dream to Angus McFergus and promised a great victory over the English. On the day of the battle a white cross appeared in the sky, and Angus was victorious. This happened at the Battle of Athelstaneford, and is the reason why the flag is blue (for the sky) with a white cross.

The first time St Andrew was officially recognised as Scotland's patron saint was at the signing of the Arbroath Declaration of independence from England. (Among those nobles who signed this was Robert the Bruce.) St Andrew's relics disappeared during the Reformation of Scotland's churches – a fragment is in St Mary's Church, Edinburgh. Scotland is one of the few countries to have one of Christ's disciples as a patron saint. Other countries are Romania, Greece and Russia – they all share St Andrew, along with various other holy persons.

2. A taste of haggis

Has anyone tasted haggis before? Encourage the group to try a little – bring it in with a brave – preferably Scottish – staff member or group member reading the poem to a haggis.

The Haggis Ceremony goes like this: the company stands and the piper leads in the haggis held aloft, followed by a person with two bottles of whisky. They march to the top table while the guests perform a slow handclap. The haggis and whisky are placed before the Chairman who, along with the chef and the piper, toasts the haggis with whisky, saying '*Slainte mhath*' (pronounced 'slan-je-va'), and the chairman then addresses the haggis thus:

To a Haggis
Fair fa' your honest, sonsie face
Great Chieftain o' the Puddin' race!
Aboon them a'ye tak your place,
Painch, tripe, or thairm:
Weel are ye wordy o' a grace
As lang's my arm.

Robert Burns

Translation:
Good luck to your honest, jolly face,
Great Chieftain of the Pudding race!
Above them all you take your place,
Paunch, tripe, or intestines:
Well are you worthy of a grace
As long as my arm.

To sample Scottish porridge, steep the oats in water earlier in the morning and microwave for one minute, stir, then 20–30 seconds more...sprinkle with salt – the Scottish way!

3. The poetry of Robbie Burns

Perhaps a member of the group would like to read one of the following poems:

To a Louse
His spindle shank a guid whip-lash
His nieve a nit
O wad some Pow'r the giftie gie us
To see ourselves as others see us!
It wad frae mony a blunder free us
And foolish notion.

Robert Burns

NB 'nieve' is offspring.

A Red, Red Rose
My luve is like a red, red rose
That's newly sprung in June.
My luve is like the melody
That's sweetly played in tune.

As fair thou art, my bonnie lass,
So deep in luve am I,
And I will luve thee still, my dear,
Till a' the seas gang dry.

Till a' the seas gang dry, my dear,
And the rocks melt wi' the sun:
And I will luve thee still, my dear,
While the sands o' life shall run.

And fare thee weel, my only luve,
And fare thee weel a while!
And I will come again, my luve,
Thou' it were ten thousand mile.

Robert Burns

4. Scottish quiz

(based on *Mental Aerobics* page 233)

Divide the group into two teams named after clans of the group's choice. One person in each team to write down the answers, then exchange to mark them.

1. What is the no man's land between England and Scotland called...the Borders
2. What is the purple, shrubby bush growing on the moors...heather
3. What is a 'crofter'...a peasant farmer
4. What is another name for Scotland...Caledonia
5. What are the most famous Scottish hills known as...the Highlands
6. Who wrote *Ivanhoe*?...Sir Walter Scott
7. Name the famous Scottish estuary near Edinburgh...Firth of Forth
8. Name a famous Scottish Presbyterian minister...John Knox
9. Where did Mary, Queen of Scots live?...Holyrood Palace
10. Name the group of islands off the west coast of Scotland...Hebrides
11. What is the capital of Scotland?...Edinburgh
12. What is the largest city?...Glasgow

13. What is the language of the Scottish highlands?...Gaelic
14. What is the pouch worn at the front of the kilt called?...sporran
15. What do Scots eat for breakfast?...porridge
16. What is the nickname of the famous monster?...Nessie
17. What sport uses a heavy pole?...caber tossing
18. Name the Scottish national instrument...bagpipes
19. When is Burns' Night?...25 January
20. Name two Scottish dances...Highland fling, sword dance, Gay Gordons
21. The small breed of ponies associated with Scotland...Shetland
22. The Scottish headgear is...a bonnet or tam-o'-shanter
23. What is supposed to be worn under the kilt?...nothing
24. The alcoholic drink of Scotland... whisky
25. The non-alcoholic drink of Scotland...Irn Bru
26. What does Mac or Mc mean?...son of
27. A famous wedding venue...the blacksmith's forge at Gretna Green
28. What are neeps?...turnips
29. What is a kirk?...church
30. A Scottish heavy horse...Clydesdale
31. Name of a Scottish soup – made from...cock o' leekie
32. What is St Andrews famous for?...a golf course and a university
33. What fuel is dug from the moors?...peat
34. A grassy, shaded area or valley...glen
35. The famous Shakespearian play that is bad luck for actors to mention...*Macbeth*
36. What is a *'ceilidh'*?...festival celebrating Gaelic dances and art
37. What is the famous shopping street in Edinburgh?...Princes Street
38. What is the famous military celebration?...the Edinburgh Tattoo
39. What did the Germans call the Scots in the war?...the Ladies from Hell
40. Where did the Campbells behave with such infamy?...Glen Coe
41. The first king of Scotland?...Robert the Bruce
42. The pin on the kilt is...a cairngorm
43. The two most famous Scottish football teams...Celtic and Rangers
44. The battle between Bonnie Prince Charlie and George II was...Culloden, 1746
45. Which Royal went to St Andrews' University?...Prince William

If the answers generate group discussion or holiday memories, encourage the chat.

5. See how many words can be made from: TAM-O'-SHANTER.

Week 4 – Animals in winter

Equipment: flipchart, pens, paper, hazelnuts, three paper cups or identical eggcups, small table, copies of the picture quiz (on page 27).

1. Reminiscence and discussion

Talk with the group about what happens to animals at this time, how they prepare for winter – grow thicker fur, store up fat on their bodies over summer to prepare for hibernation, some mass together for warmth (wrens), hide food stores (squirrels). Ask the group to name as many animals as they can that hibernate (hedgehogs, bears – who often give birth to their cubs when hibernating – tortoises, some insects such as ladybirds and peacock butterflies). NB Squirrels don't fully hibernate – they slow down and use their food stores to tide them over...if they can remember where they hid them!

Did anyone own a tortoise? What happened to it in winter? Does the group remember the *Blue Peter* tortoise being put away to hibernate?

Does anyone feed the birds? What do they give the birds to eat? Has anyone got any stories about the antics of the squirrels on the bird table? Does the group think the warmer winters are having an effect on animals that hibernate?

Ask how they or their parents prepared for wintertime...did they make jams? Pickles? Bottle fruit and vegetables from the garden? Store apples and pears on special shelves? String onions? Salt meat? Tell how the Romans used to fatten dormice in special jars to provide some meat for hard times. Dovecotes were also used as a source of fresh meat. In many countries meat is dried to enable it to be kept for a long time – ask if anyone has tried dried meat – and in freezing climates meat is stored in ice. Ask the group what is the strangest meat they have eaten.

Did anyone live on a farm? How did they prepare for winter? Store root vegetables? Feed for the animals? Silage or hay? Did they bring the animals inside? If hill farmers – how did they get the sheep down off the hills? Did the animals ever go hungry in the severe winters of long ago? How do their pets behave during the cold weather? Do some of them wear coats/boots? Do they struggle to get them to go out?

2. 'Jumbled animals' picture quiz

If possible show the picture on page 27 on an overhead projector but also give everyone a copy of the picture, and ask each person to identify an animal, say if it is British and if it hibernates. Ask them to actually pinpoint the animal, e.g. 'top righthand corner, on top of the camel', 'middle of the picture, next to the skunk's tail'.

The less complicated picture on page 28 can be substituted.

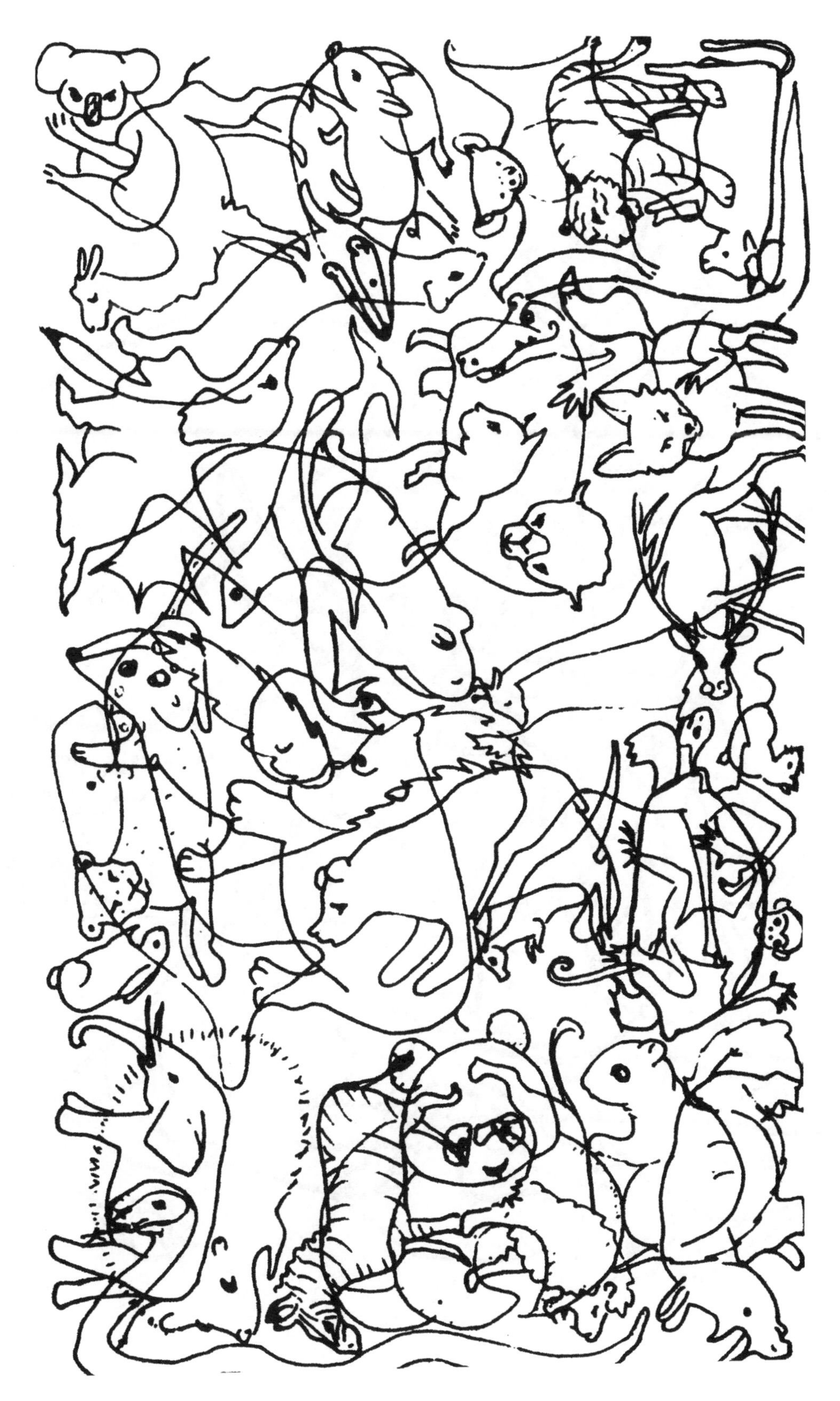

Answers: Cow, elephant, leopard, badger, pig, giraffe, zebra, monkey, sheep, rhino, stoat, mouse, dog, seal, fox, frog, tortoise, bat, camel, panda, hippo, snake, bear, skunk, lion, tiger, rabbit, whale, stag, squirrel, hedgehog, koala, cat, kangaroo, crocodile

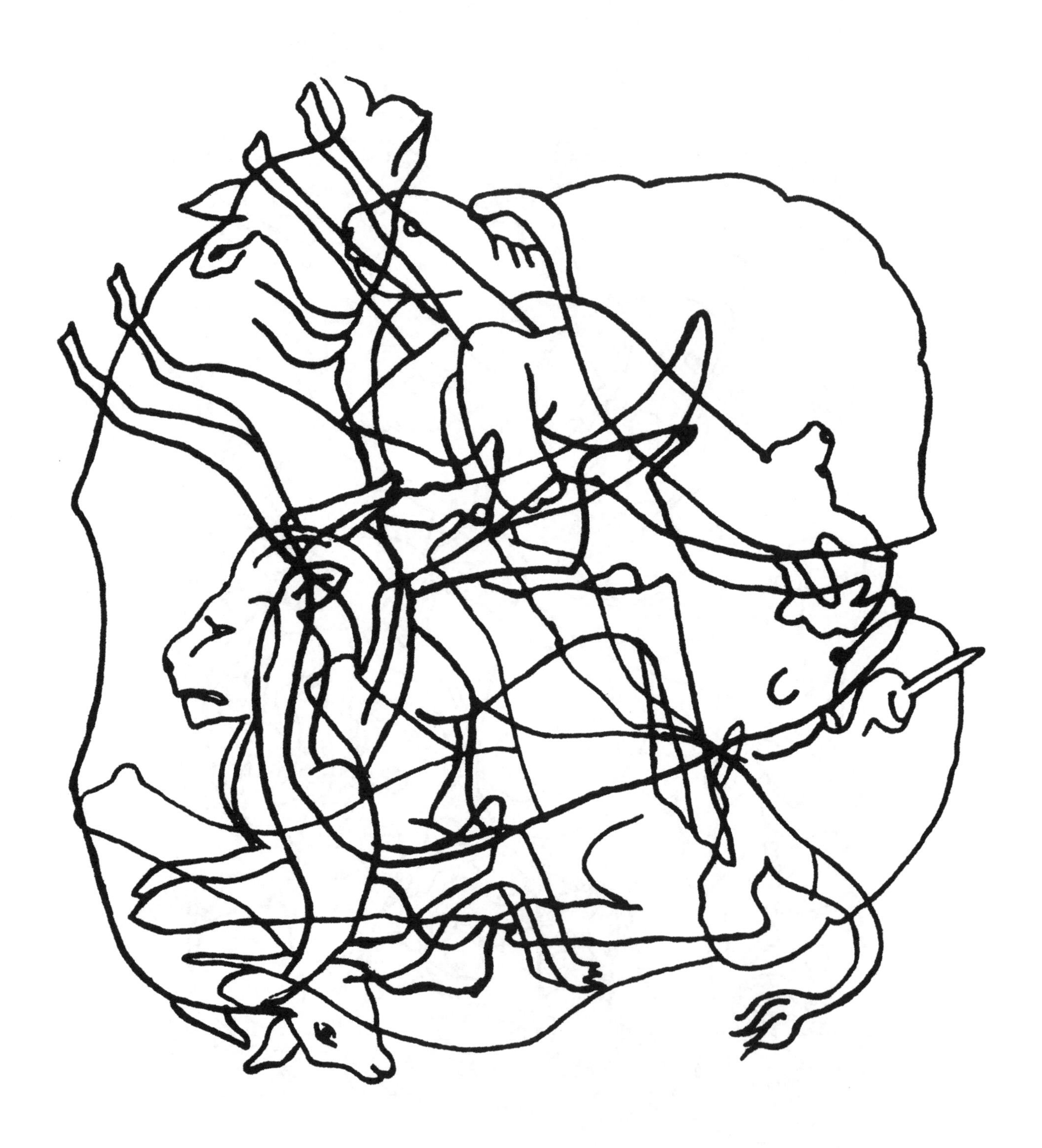

Answers: Elephant, lion, tortoise, kangaroo, deer, polar bear, rhino

3. Animal metaphors

(based on *More Mental Aerobics* page 104)

Read out the first part of the saying for the group to complete either individually or as a group.

1. As busy as…a bee
2. As fat as…a pig
3. As wise as…an owl
4. As sly as…a fox
5. As bold as…a lion
6. As stubborn as…a mule
7. As free as…a bird
8. As slow as…a tortoise
9. As small as…a mouse
10. As proud as…a peacock
11. As cold as…a fish
12. As weak as…a kitten
13. As hungry as…a horse
14. As cheeky as…a monkey
15. As tall as…a giraffe
16. As slow as…a snail
17. As big as…an elephant
18. As strong as…an ox
19. As sleek as…a cat
20. As silly as…a goose
21. As meek as…a lamb
22. As cunning as…a box of monkeys
23. As ancient as…a dinosaur
24. As quiet as…a mouse
25. As mad as…a bull (or March hare)
26. As blind as…a bat
27. As happy as…a lark
28. As happy as a dog with…two tails

Ask the group for more.

4. Find the hazelnut!

On the small table have the three cups in a row, place one hazelnut under a cup and ask each person in turn to watch as the cups are quickly shuffled around, then identify the cup the nut is under. If correct, they get another try – three times correct, and they win the nut!

5. Animal quiz

Use the flipchart to write the answers, as there may be more than one
What animals:

1. Carry their young in a pouch?…kangaroos, wallabies
2. Have stripes?…tigers, zebras, skunks
3. Have bushy tails?…squirrels
4. Sleep by day upside-down?…bats

5. Live mostly in trees?...apes, monkeys, birds
6. Have very long necks?...giraffes
7. Are called 'ships of the desert'?...camels
8. Have bodies covered in spines?...hedgehogs, porcupines
9. Have one or two humps on their backs?...camels (To tell the difference between Dromedaries (one hump) and Bactrians (two humps) turn the initial capital letter on its side.)
10. Like to build dams?...beavers
11. Are called 'man's best friend'...dogs?
12. Are the King of the Beasts?...lions
13. Kill snakes?...mongooses
14. Have cloven hooves?...cows, deer, sheep, goats
15. Can be ridden?...horses, donkeys', camels
16. Have retractable claws?...cats
17. Live in the sea?...whales, dolphins, seals, walrus
18. Have tusks?...walrus, elephans, wild boars
19. Only eat bamboo shoots?...pandas
20. Roll in a ball for protection?...hedgehogs

6. See how many words can be made from: HIBERNATION.

Activities for February

Week 1 – 'When we made our own fun'

Equipment: flipchart, paper, pens, dominoes, marbles, yo-yo, tiddlywinks, skipping rope; card games such as Old Maid, Donkey, Snap, Happy Families; board games – Ludo, Monopoly, Cluedo, Snakes and Ladders; crossword puzzles; enlarged copies of grids for 'Battleships' (page 32) and 'Squares' (page 33).

1. Reminiscence and discussion

Talk with the group about how they used to pass the long winter evenings when they were young. What games did they play? What kind of hobbies did they have? Do they still pursue them now? Would they like to? Do they need assistance to do this? Does anyone have a particular hobby or pastime now? Make a list on the flipchart…it will be amazing to see the range of talent in the room! Ask people to bring in samples of their work, e.g. knitting, embroidery, marquetry, painting, etc. What sort of hobbies did their parents have? Were they allowed to do these things on Sundays? If not, what were they allowed to do? What sort of things do their children and grandchildren do? Would they have liked to try these hobbies?

2. Games and pastimes challenge

Ask the group if they would like a trip down Memory Lane and would be happy to join in some of the old games.

NOUGHTS AND CROSSES

Give everyone a piece of paper and a pen and ask them to play ten games with the person on either side of them. Perhaps there could be a play-off between the best players.

BATTLESHIPS

See if any of the group remember how to play 'Battleships'. In pairs, starting with a copy of the grid for each person, the players draw their ships over a grid by colouring in squares:

- 5 cruisers on each of 3 squares
- 3 destroyers on each of 4 squares
- 1 battleship on each of 5 squares.

In turn, they pick a square (say, B8), and if their opponent has a ship, or part of a ship, on that square, he or she must admit to being bombed – and be *honest*!

	A	B	C	D	E	F	G	H	I	J
1										
2										
3										
4										
5										
6										
7										
8										
9										
10										

SQUARES

Still in pairs, they may like to play 'Squares'. Using the grid of dots, they take it in turns to draw a line from one dot to the next, the object being to form a square. If the line they draw completes the box, they can claim it by putting their initials in it. The winner is the person who has the most squares.

3. Card games

Have the group split into fours to play each card game. Move on to the next game after completing each one, until all have been played.

- Snap
- Old Maid
- Donkey
- Beggar my Neighbour.

4. Board games

- Ludo
- Monopoly
- Snakes and Ladders
- Cluedo

If there is a surplus number of people in the group, those people could play Patience or Clock patience until they can swap into a foursome.

5. Picture consequences

Come back into the whole group to play. Give everyone a narrow strip of paper, then ask everyone to draw the head of a person or an animal, leaving a longish neck. They each then fold their paper so that just the lines of the neck are showing, and pass it to the person on their right. Everyone then draws a body to the waist, including arms, then folds their paper so that the edge of the waist is showing and again passes it on to their right. Everyone next draws a pair of legs, then completely folds the paper and passes it on to their right. In turn, everyone fully opens a paper to expose the (hopefully) funny drawings, and show each in turn to everyone. Do this a few times, if going well. If people are enjoying this, play:

6. Consequences

Each person has a narrow piece of paper and writes a girl's name, then folds paper and passes to right. They then write a boy's name, which is likewise passed on. They next write where they met, fold and pass on; then what *she* said, fold and pass on; then what *he* said, fold and pass on; and finally, the consequence of this meeting, which is also folded and passed to the right. In turn, each person reads theirs as a story, e.g., 'Mary Smith met Tommy Steele in or at 10, Downing Street, she said, "You look bigger on TV." He said, "Is that your own hair?" and the consequence, was they signed a prenuptial agreement…'

7. 'I Spy'

Play as a whole group and make sure each person has a go, even if they don't guess correctly.

8. Make a paper aeroplane and fly it!

Give everyone a square of paper. The furthest flight wins a jelly baby.

Week 2 – St Valentine's Day

Equipment: flipchart, paper, pens, 'Love Heart' sweeties, heart-shaped cards.

1. Reminiscence and discussion

Talk with the group about St Valentine's Day in the past. It only began in Victorian times and is now a billion-dollar industry all over the world. Did members of the group send cards? Can they remember the first one they received? Did they know who sent it? Did they stay with their first love? When they got married did they still send a Valentine card, and do they even now? Did anyone send or receive a special gift on this day? What? What does the group feel are romantic gifts? Did anyone compose a verse to go with their Valentine? Was it 'Roses are red, violets are blue, Sugar is sweet and so are you'? can they recall their own compositions? Do they remember the codes they used on the back of envelopes to their lover? S.W.A.L.K. was very popular. Can they remember its meaning – (Sealed With a Loving Kiss)? B.O.L.T.O.P (Better on Lips Than on Paper) was another. Any more?

Does the group know why 14 February is the date to celebrate love? Traditionally it is the birds' wedding day! Also, it is St Valentine's Day. Valentine was a Roman priest executed for marrying lovers against the wishes of the Emperor Claudius II.

The oldest Valentine card dates from the fifteenth century and is in the British museum. The most expensive Valentine's Day card was sent by Aristotle Onassis to Maria Callas – a solid gold card studded with diamonds, wrapped in a mink coat.

Does the group know any of the superstitions related to this day? For example, that you will marry the first person you see on Valentine's Day? Or, if a woman sees a robin, she will marry a sailor, if a sparrow, it will be a poor man, but if a goldfinch, she will marry a millionaire.

There was a famous massacre on this day in 1929, when the notorious gangster Al Capone and his men gunned down a rival gang. (Does anyone remember how Capone was finally caught? It was for non-payment of income tax.)

2. Love hearts

Give everyone a love heart and ask each in turn to read the message. Give out the cardboard heart shapes and pens and ask everyone to make their own 'love heart'. See if they are more romantic than Swizzel's sweetie ones.

3. Heart quiz

(based on *Mental Aerobics* page 257)

Each answer contains the word 'heart'.

1. Overwhelming unhappiness...heartbreak
2. Too much stomach acid...heartburn
3. A card suit...hearts
4. Sorrow or distress...heartache
5. Myocardial infarction...heart attack

14. Something sincere and deep...heartfelt
15. Too kind...soft-hearted
16. Carpet in front of the fire...hearthrug
17. Word meaning 'to encourage'...hearten
18. Two song titles...'Heart of my Heart', 'Heartbreak Hotel', and any others

6. Someone we have a crush on...heartthrob
7. A pet name...sweetheart
8. Lacking in courage...fainthearted
9. The tart thief...Knave of Hearts
10. The pulsing of the heart...heartbeat
11. An unfaithful lover...heartbreaker
12. Indifferent to others' feelings...cold-hearted
13. Brother of King John...Richard the Lionheart
19. An American medal...Purple Heart
20. A tart maker...Queen of Hearts
21. To do something with gusto...heartily
22. Machine used in heart operations...heart–lung machine
23. Someone we love tenderly pulls at these...heartstrings
24. Very upset and sad...heavy-hearted
25. Large as in breakfast, loud as in laughter...hearty
26. Without feeling...stony-hearted

4. 'I love my love'

Beginning with the letter 'A' and working through the alphabet, each group member in turn thinks of an appropriate adjective, a person's name (*male* for a female group member, *female* for a male group member) and a place, all beginning with the same letter, and speaks the whole sentence. For example:

I love my love because he is Adorable.

His name is Albert.

He lives in Accrington.

Then the next person does the same with the next letter of the alphabet – for example:

I love my love because she is Blonde.

Her name is Barbara.

She lives in Bootle.

– and so on...

5. Famous couples

(from *Mental Aerobics* page 260)

Give the name of one of a pair and ask the group to name the other.

Romeo – Juliet

Samson – Delilah

Napoleon – Josephine

Antony – Cleopatra

William – Mary

Jack – Jill

Adam – Eve
Victoria – Albert
Peter Pan – Wendy
Robin Hood – Maid Marian
Bonnie – Clyde
Nelson – Lady Hamilton
J.F.K. – Jackie Kennedy
Elizabeth Taylor – Richard Burton
William Shakespeare – Anne Hathaway
Othello – Desdemona
Elizabeth Browning – Robert Browning
Sonny – Cher
Helen of Troy – Paris
Punch – Judy
Margaret Thatcher – Dennis
Winston – Clementine
Vera Duckworth – Jack
Paul Daniels – Debbie McGee
Charles – Camilla
Fred Astaire – Ginger Rogers
Donald Duck – Daisy
Grace Kelly – Prince Rainier
Popeye – Olive Oyl
Guinevere – King Arthur
Edward VIII – Mrs Simpson
Hitler – Eva Braun
Mary – Joseph
John Lennon – Yoko Ono
Ronald Reagan – Nancy
Humphrey Bogart – Lauren Bacall
Cinderella – Prince Charming
Mickey Mouse – Minnie Mouse
Tony Blair – Cherie
Richard – Judy
Troilus – Cressida

6. Valentine mix

(based on *Mental Aerobics* page 259)

Write anagrams on the flipchart and ask the group to write the answers on paper supplied.

PUDIC	cupid	NOWOS	swoon
OOCCHETAL	chocolate	YFBDOENIR	boyfriend
SWROELF	flowers	MESOOTW	twosome
SKSI	kiss	BEALSPIANRE	inseparable
RTOUCHIPS	courtship	TOQEBUU	bouquet
TEWESATREH	sweetheart	YPPHA	happy
VOLE	love	DRE SEORS	red roses
SORARW	arrows	LPSI	lips
BIBONRS	ribbons	NAITS TELINAVNE	Saint Valentine

7. Who in all the world or in history would they most like to send a red rose to?

– and *to whom would they send a raspberry?* List replies on the flipchart.

Week 3 – Chinese New Year

Equipment: flipchart, paper, scissors, sticky tape, pens, selection of different Chinese teas to try – green tea, jasmine tea, Lapsang souchong – prawn crackers or fortune cookies, chopsticks, copies of calendar/animal charts on pages 39–40.

1. Reminiscence and discussion

Talk about China with the group. Has anyone been there? Anyone been to Hong Kong? What did they think about it? Has anyone been to the Chinatown areas of the big cities such as Manchester? Can anyone think of anything relating to Chinese culture? Some prompts:

- The binding of girl children's feet – to prove they were aristocratic and unable to work in the fields. Can people think of the film that told how Gladys Hailwood went to China on a mission to stop this practice – (*Inn of the Sixth Happiness*)? Has anyone seen the tiny Chinese women's shoes that are sometimes displayed in the curio cabinets of stately homes?
- What is the name of the special means of transport that used to be manpowered but now can be motorised or bicycle powered? (Rickshaw)
- What kind of boats do the Chinese Boat People live their whole lives on? (Sampans)
- Can the group remember the name of the drug that caused the savage war in the eighteenth century? (Opium)
- What luxurious material came to us from China? (Silk.) Does the group know how it is made? (The cocoons of silkworms are soaked in hot water and a single thread of silk about a mile long is collected and woven into beautiful garments.) What do the silkworms eat? (Mulberry leaves.) King James I tried to start a silk industry in England but he grew the wrong type of mulberry trees, so it failed.
- Has the group heard of the 'Little Emperors' of China? There is a government directive stating the people can only have one child per family (to reduce the soaring population). People are fined if they have more, and so these single children become totally spoiled. There is also the horrendous practice in the rural area of allowing girl babies to die, as girls are seen as worthless, but boys can work the land and help support their parents in old age. This has caused an imbalance in the sexes, and now some young men have no one to marry.

- Ask the group if they can remember the Cultural Revolution. What was the name of the Mao's book? (Chairman Mao's *Little Red Book*.) Mao destroyed a whole generation of intellectuals by making them leave university and go to work on the land.
- Can anyone remember the bravery of the unknown rebel who faced the tanks on Tiananmen Square in Beijing?
- Do people think of the capital as 'Peking' or 'Beijing'? Did they enjoy the Olympic Games? What about the pollution – did it affect the athletes?

Using the flipchart, write down all the Chinese-related things the group can list – for example, gunpowder, fireworks, silk, Great Wall of China, chopsticks, tea, jasmine, opium poppies, takeaway meals, paddy-fields, jade, dragons, Pekinese dogs, gambling, Aladdin, Wishee-Washee, Chinese laundry, Charlie Chan (detective), Tiger Lily (Rupert Bear's friend), kites. Does anyone remember the nursery rhyme 'Chin Chin China man, How much are your geese?'?

2. Chinese calendar

Chinese years are named after one of twelve animals. Each animal is said to have its own personality and emotions, and people born in that year are said to be like the animal it is named for.

Find out which animal you are with the following chart.

Year of the:										
RAT	1900	1912	1924	1936	1948	1960	1972	1984	1996	2008
OX	1901	1913	1925	1937	1949	1961	1973	1985	1997	2009
TIGER	1902	1914	1926	1938	1950	1962	1974	1986	1998	2010
RABBIT	1903	1915	1927	1939	1951	1963	1975	1987	1999	2011
DRAGON	1904	1916	1928	1940	1952	1964	1976	1988	2000	2012
SNAKE	1905	1917	1929	1941	1953	1965	1977	1989	2001	2013
HORSE	1906	1918	1930	1942	1954	1966	1978	1990	2002	2014
RAM	1907	1919	1931	1943	1955	1967	1979	1991	2003	2015
MONKEY	1908	1920	1932	1944	1956	1968	1980	1992	2004	2016
ROOSTER	1909	1921	1933	1945	1957	1969	1981	1993	2005	2017
DOG	1910	1922	1934	1946	1958	1970	1982	1994	2006	2018
PIG	1911	1923	1935	1947	1959	1971	1983	1995	2007	2019

ANIMAL CHARACTERISTICS

Are you like your year animal?

RAT	Cheerful, charming, welcome everywhere. Craves excitement and is easily bored.
OX	Hard-working and patient. Can be shy or difficult; self-reliant.
TIGER	Forceful personality, adventurous and confident. Sees all sides of a problem but not the answer.
RABBIT	Home lover, peaceable and sociable. Often shy and secretive.
DRAGON	Strong personality. Loves freedom, hates routine. Popular and generous but can be inconsistent.
SNAKE	Sensitive with a strong sense of responsibility, charming, with well-developed sense of humour. Sometimes selfish and likes to hoard money.
HORSE	Hard-working, admirable, ambitious, careful with money, but likes to play hard.
RAM	Gentle and caring, achieves by kindness, loves beautiful things and has strong family feelings.
MONKEY	Charming, cheeky and clever, often with little respect for authority, creative and successful in most things, especially business.
ROOSTER	Faithful to family and friends, organised, punctual and hard-working – can be arrogant in giving unasked-for advice.
DOG	Loyal, caring, with a fearless streak, hates injustice and needs to learn more patience when trying to change things.
PIG	Peace-loving, trusting, strong and straightforward. Likes a quiet life, makes a good leader but prefers to be a team member.

3. Chop-chop

Has the group tried Chinese food? What are their favourites? Can anyone use chopsticks? In turn, each person tries to pick up a prawn cracker – and eat it – with chopsticks.

4. Superstitions

The Chinese believe in good and bad luck and have many superstitions. Superstitions are defined as an irrational belief in charms and omens, coupled with a dread of the supernatural. Can the group list any of their own superstitions, or any they have heard of? Does anyone have a 'lucky' rabbit's foot? A lucky pair of shoes? A lucky number or colour? Do they have a ritual they must complete before doing something, like the famous sportsmen? Some examples:

- Friday 13th is thought to be unlucky.
- To move house on a Friday is unlucky – 'Friday flit, short sit'.
- To step on a crack in the pavement is unlucky. (How many avoided this before a spelling/maths test at school?)
- To bring May blossom into the house is unlucky.
- Red and white flowers together are avoided on hospital wards as unlucky – they are reminiscent of blood and bandages.
- An albatross is an unlucky omen if it lands on your boat.
- Crossed knives are portents of a quarrel.
- If your clothes are inside-out or back-to-front, do not change them, or you will change your luck.
- If your right palm itches, it means cash – 'right to receive, left to leave'.
- First day of the month, either say 'white rabbits' or 'pinch, punch, first of the month'.
- Touch wood to avert bad luck.
- Don't walk under a ladder.
- On seeing a magpie, you must say 'Good morning/afternoon, Mr Magpie' to stop the bad luck.
- Also on seeing magpies: 'one for sorrow, two for joy, three for a girl, four for a boy'.
- Finding a four-leaved clover is very lucky.
- White heather is lucky.
- If you spill salt, throw a pinch over your left shoulder into the devil's eye and stop bad luck.
- If you break a mirror you will have seven years' bad luck.
- The bride must wear 'something borrowed, something blue, something old, something new'.
- A chimneysweep at the wedding brings good luck.
- 'Marry in May and rue the day.'
- Black cats are lucky.
- Brides should not wear pearls, as 'pearls are for tears'.
- 'Happy the bride the sun shines on.'
- Horseshoes are lucky if hung upwards (u) but the luck runs out if they are hung down (n).
- It is unlucky to come in one door and out of another – it means you won't be returning.
- If a money spider crosses your palm, you will get some money.

5. Chinese quiz

(based on *Mental Aerobics* page 195)

Ask the group in general. Some assistance may be needed for the more difficult questions.

1. Name two rivers in China...the Yellow River, the Yangtze
2. Where is rice grown?...paddyfields
3. What are the Chinese eating implements called?...chopsticks
4. Name two Chinese dynasties....any of these: Ming, Tang, Manchu, Shang
5. What is the Chinese way of frying meat and vegetables in oil called?...stir-fry
6. Name the famous Chinese soup...bird's nest
7. What lies at the heart of Beijing?...the Forbidden City
8. What in China is said to be seen from outer space?... the Great Wall
9. What was the ancient trade route called?...the Silk Road
10. Who is China's most famous chairman?...Mao Tse Tung
11. Name two Chinese vegetables...water chestnuts, beansprouts, bamboo shoots
12. What is the correct name of modern China?...People's Republic of China
13. What is opium obtained from?...poppies
14. What is the largest city in China?...Shanghai
15. What mythical animal is always in Chinese parades?...dragon
16. What ancient adding machine did the Chinese invent?...abacus
17. How do the Chinese ward off evil spirits?...set off firecrackers
18. What is the puller of a rickshaw and a paddyfield worker called?...coolie
19. When did the Cultural Revolution occur?...1966–1976
20. What is China's precious stone?...jade
21. What is China's most popular means of transport?...bicycle
22. What is Zhezhi (the predecessor of origami)?...the art of folding paper
23. What is the Chinese game similar to chess called?...Mah-jong
24. What ancient martial art is practised by young and old in China?...T'ai Chi
25. Who was the famous Chinese Nationalist Leader?...Chiang Kai-Shek
26. What is China's favourite snack?...sunflower seeds
27. What is China's favourite flower?...chrysthanthemum
28. What flavouring is used most often in Chinese food?...monosodium glutamate
29. Name the thirteenth-century explorer of China...Marco Polo
30. Name three animals used to denote years in the Chinese calendar...(see pages 39–40)

6. Paper art

Give everyone a piece of paper, scissors and sticky tape and ask them to make either a Chinese lantern or a coolie hat, ready to celebrate the Chinese New Year.

CHINESE NEW YEAR

In all the towns and villages, coloured banners and lanterns decorate the houses, the houses are thoroughly cleaned and decorated with flowers to honour the kitchen god, food is prepared, and debts paid off. Fireworks are set off and new clothes are worn to symbolise discarding the old year and its misfortunes, gifts are given to family and friends. Special rice cakes and kumquats (for prosperity) and red paper packets containing money are given by married couples to children and unmarried family and friends. Parades with firecrackers, gongs and drums, performing lions and dragon dances go through the streets collecting the red money packets, and fruit and vegetables are hung from the shops in hope of good fortune. The celebrations end with the Lantern Festival when the children parade through the streets with lighted lanterns.

7. 'KUNG HAY FAT CHOY'

This is the Cantonese way of greeting revellers, and means 'May you prosper'. How many words can be made from this greeting? And can everyone say it?

Whilst this activity is going on, pass round different teas to try, and give each person a fortune cookie if possible.

Week 4 – Planting for spring

Equipment: flipchart, pens, paper, dice, video *The Land Girls* (for later viewing if requested), selection of bulbs, compost and pots, copies of word search chart on page 47.

1. Reminiscence and discussion

Talk with the group about gardens they may have had in the past. Did they have their own patch when they were a child? What plants did they grow? Anyone remember growing cress on a facecloth? Did they have any weird plants such as Venus' flytrap?

Did anyone have an allotment? What vegetables did they grow? Do any of the group remember 'dig for victory' in the War? Because of food rationing many open spaces, parks, etc. were given over to food production.

Was anyone in the Land Army, or does the group remember anyone being in the Land Army? Has anyone seen the video? Would they like to?

Did anyone enter the local Flower and Produce Show? Did they have prizewinning exhibits? What was the secret of their success? Any tips on producing giant onions, marrows, sunflowers? What are the group's favourite flowers and vegetables? Ask each person and note their answers on the flipchart. It may be interesting to see how similar they are, and if men and women have different preferences.

Talk about the fresh taste of homegrown tomatoes and strawberries. Does anyone still grow a few salad crops or vegetables or flowers? Do they have a windowbox if in a flat? Or just grow plants on their windowsills? Do people enjoy the gardening programmes on TV? Who is their favourite presenter? Which kind of programme do they prefer – the garden makeover, or the factual type that gives hints and shows experts' gardens?

Discuss the properties of plants. Does anyone remember old remedies using plants? (*Comfrey* for bruises, *lavender* for headache and to scent underwear drawers, *rue* to keep away flies, *dock leaves* for nettle stings, *rosewater* made from rose petals, *pot marigolds* planted as a companion plant to stop pests attacking crops, *cucumber* slices on tired eyes, *camomile* lawns to soothe and relax, *feverfew* for headaches.)

Ask the group for tips on getting rid of pests, especially slugs – maybe the group could research the different methods later in the year to see which is the most successful. (Make note in diary to do this.)

2. Gardening quiz

Ask each person in turn.

1. Which flower grows tall and turns to face the sun?...sunflower
2. Name the small, spade-like handtool...trowel
3. What leaves a shiny trail in the garden?...slugs and snails
4. Why do gardeners put nets over fruit?...to protect from birds
5. Which fleshy desert plant grows in the greenhouse?...cactus
6. What colour are forget-me-nots?...blue
7. When will you see snowdrops?...early spring
8. What colour are primroses?...yellow
9. What would you use to take leaves off the lawn?...rake, blower or garden vac
10. Why are flowers brightly coloured and perfumed?...to attract bees and insects
11. What is the straight row seeds are planted in called?...a drill
12. What is a dibber?...a small, pointed, wooden stick for making planting holes
13. How would you protect tender plants from frost?...use a cloche/garden floss
14. What is another name for an aphid?...greenfly
15. What is a perennial?...a plant that flowers every year
16. What is the art of dwarfing trees called?...bonsai
17. What caused the Potato Famine in Ireland?...potato blight
18. What are fennel, basil and marjoram?...herbs
19. What are clematis and wisteria?...climbers

20. What is chlorophyll?...the green substance of the plant that produces its food.
21. What is the cutting out of deadwood called?...pruning
22. When is the Chelsea Flower Show held?...May
23. What type of soil do rhododendrons prefer?...acid
24. Name the opium plant...poppy
25. Peonies are commonly what colour?...red, pink
26. What are pruning tools called?...secateurs
27. What do we know *digitalis purpurea* as?...foxglove
28. What is a trellis arch with climbers on it called?...pergola
29. What temperature gives frost?...under 0° Centigrade, 32° Fahrenheit
30. Climbers, ramblers, teas and standards are all...roses
31. Anyone know the Latin name of hollyhocks?...*althaeas*
32. What is a hybrid?...the offspring of two different species or varieties
33. A plant that completes its life cycle in two years is a...biennial
34. What is the trumpet of the daffodil called?...corona
35. What is the prong of a fork known as?...a tine
36. What does the iris grow from?...a rhizome
37. What would sulphur dust cure?...fungus, mildew
38. In what would saxifrage, oxalis and edelweiss grow?...a rockery

3. Flower alphabet

(based on *More Mental Aerobics* page 297)

In turn, ask group members to give the name of a flower, in alphabetical order – they can all help if a person is stuck.

A anemone, azalea
B bluebell, buttercup
C crocus, carnation, chrysthanthemum
D daffodil, daisy, dahlia
E edelweiss
F forget-me-not, foxglove
G gardenia, geranium
H hollyhock, harebell
I iris
N narcissus
O orchid
P pink, petunia, primrose, polyanthus
Q Queen Anne's lace
R rose
S sweet pea, snowdrop, sunflower, sweet william
T tulip
U urnflower
V violet, viola

J jasmine
K kingcup
L lily, lobelia, larkspur
M marigold
W wallflower, water lily
X xanthium
Y yucca
Z zinnia

4. Flower 'Beetle'

Play in groups of four, with paper and a dice for each table. Give each person paper and pen – in turn, they shake the dice and try to draw a flower (as in the game of 'Beetle').

On the flipchart, write the values of the dice throws:

1 = nothing
2 = the flower pot
3 = stem
4 = a leaf (need two)
5 = petals (need six)
6 = flower centre

The first person to complete a drawing of a potted flower is the winner.

This game could be played by two teams named after spring flowers, where each person in turn throws the dice and the flowers are drawn by staff. The first team to complete a flower wins.

5. See how many words can be made from: HORTICULTURAL.

6. Bunch of flowers

S	V	F	C	O	W	S	L	I	P	X	W	Q	A
T	O	I	R	I	S	Y	P	P	O	P	V	B	M
O	D	A	I	S	Y	V	O	R	C	H	I	D	Q
C	H	O	N	E	Y	S	U	C	K	L	E	G	Y
K	V	R	O	S	E	G	T	R	D	S	L	J	B
W	I	L	L	I	A	M	T	E	E	W	S	L	W
E	O	S	P	R	I	M	R	O	S	E	E	G	V
B	L	U	E	B	E	L	L	S	S	E	U	Y	H
U	E	S	C	O	T	C	H	D	N	T	D	P	W
T	T	H	I	S	T	L	E	R	O	P	S	A	E
T	S	W	A	L	L	F	L	O	W	E	R	S	E
E	A	C	L	I	L	Y	H	P	E	A	T	T	D
R	A	A	Q	U	I	L	E	G	I	A	T	E	R
C	U	P	A	F	R	I	C	A	N	X	L	R	R

Can you find these hidden words?
COWSLIP, POPPY, ORCHID, ASTER, IRIS, HONEYSUCKLE, ROSE, SWEET WILLIAM, LILY, PRIMROSE, BLUEBELLS, WALL FLOWER, AQULIEGIA, BUTTER CUP, AFRICAN VIOLETS, SCOTCH THISTLE, DAISY, PEAT.

7. Plant bulbs if available.

Activities for March

Week 1 – St David's Day and Wales

Equipment: flipchart, paper, pens, tourist information on Wales. To sample if possible: Welsh rarebit, bara brith, laverbread, Welsh cakes. Copies of the 'Ds' quiz on page 50, copies of 'It's all Welsh to me' (page 51).

1. Reminiscence and discussion

Ask if the group knows the date of St David's Day (1 March). Ask if they have visited Wales. Where did they go? Did they stay or just have a day trip? Was it in a caravan? a tent? B&B, hotel, or rented cottage? Make a list of as many places in Wales as they can think of...with spellings if possible. Can anyone list the castles? (Flint, Denbigh, Rhuddlan, Conwy, Beaumaris, Dolwyddelan, Dolbadarn, Caernarvon, Harlech, Criccieth, Cilgerran, Kidwelly, Carreg Cennen.)

Ask the group what the emblems of Wales are (leek, daffodil and harp).

St David died on 1 March 589 AD and was so respected that pilgrims said two pilgrimages to St David's was worth one to Rome!

The Welsh have retained more of their Celtic culture than most of the British Isles and this has led to a strong sense of national identity. Does anyone know the political party of Wales (Plaid Cymru)? They are now self-governing – does the group think England should be?

The Welsh are famous singers, can the group name the special celebration of song and poetry the Welsh hold (Eisteddfod)?

Mining is one of the most famous industries and the minerals mined are

- **coal** – does the group remember the terrible landslide at Aberfan when the school was engulfed by the slagheap?
- **gold** – jewellery worn by Welsh princes denoted their rank. Today the wedding rings of royal brides are made from this.
- **slate** – quarries are still worked. The children's cartoon train Ivor the Engine worked the Welsh slate mines.

Has anyone been to Portmerion? What is it famous for? (*The Prisoner* was filmed here; and special pottery.)

2. Famous Davids quiz

Ask the group in general:

1. Patron saint of Wales...St David
2. Son of Princess Margaret...Viscount David Lindley
3. Magician with a bald head – from the old days!...David Nixon
4. Former British prime minister...David Lloyd George
5. A former showjumper (new one sweeps clean)...David Broome
6. Played Hutch in *Starsky and Hutch*...David Soul
7. Former British Olympic athlete (also a board used on nails)...David Emery
8. TV presenter – a cold Sir!...David Frost
9. Footballer who can 'bend it'...David Beckham
10. Sports commentator (*Question of Sport* man)...David Coleman
11. *Juke Box Jury* presenter...David Jacobs
12. Olympic swimmer...David Wilkie
13. *Only Fools and Horses, A Touch of Frost, Open All Hours* star...David Jason
14. Scottish Grand Prix driver...David Coulthard
15. Former Lib Dem leader...David Steele
16. Crooner from the old days...David Whitfield
17. British tennis player...David Lloyd
18. A Dickens novel...*David Copperfield*
19. American illusionist also...David Copperfield
20. Cricketer like the Welsh peninsula...David Gower
21. Photographer from the sixties...David Bailey
22. Brother of Jonathan, son of Richard...David Dimbleby
23. Pop star with a county name...David Essex
24. Was a runner, now presents sport...David Moorcroft
25. Blind politician...David Blunkett
26. Zoologist with a beard...David Bellamy
27. Romantic old-time film star...David Niven
28. Stanley presumed to meet him in Africa...David Livingstone
29. Brother of Richard, presenter of wildlife programmes...David Attenborough
30. Former footballer and TV presenter with odd beliefs...David Ike

3. Find all the 'D' words

After all the Davids, how many words begin with 'D' in the picture?

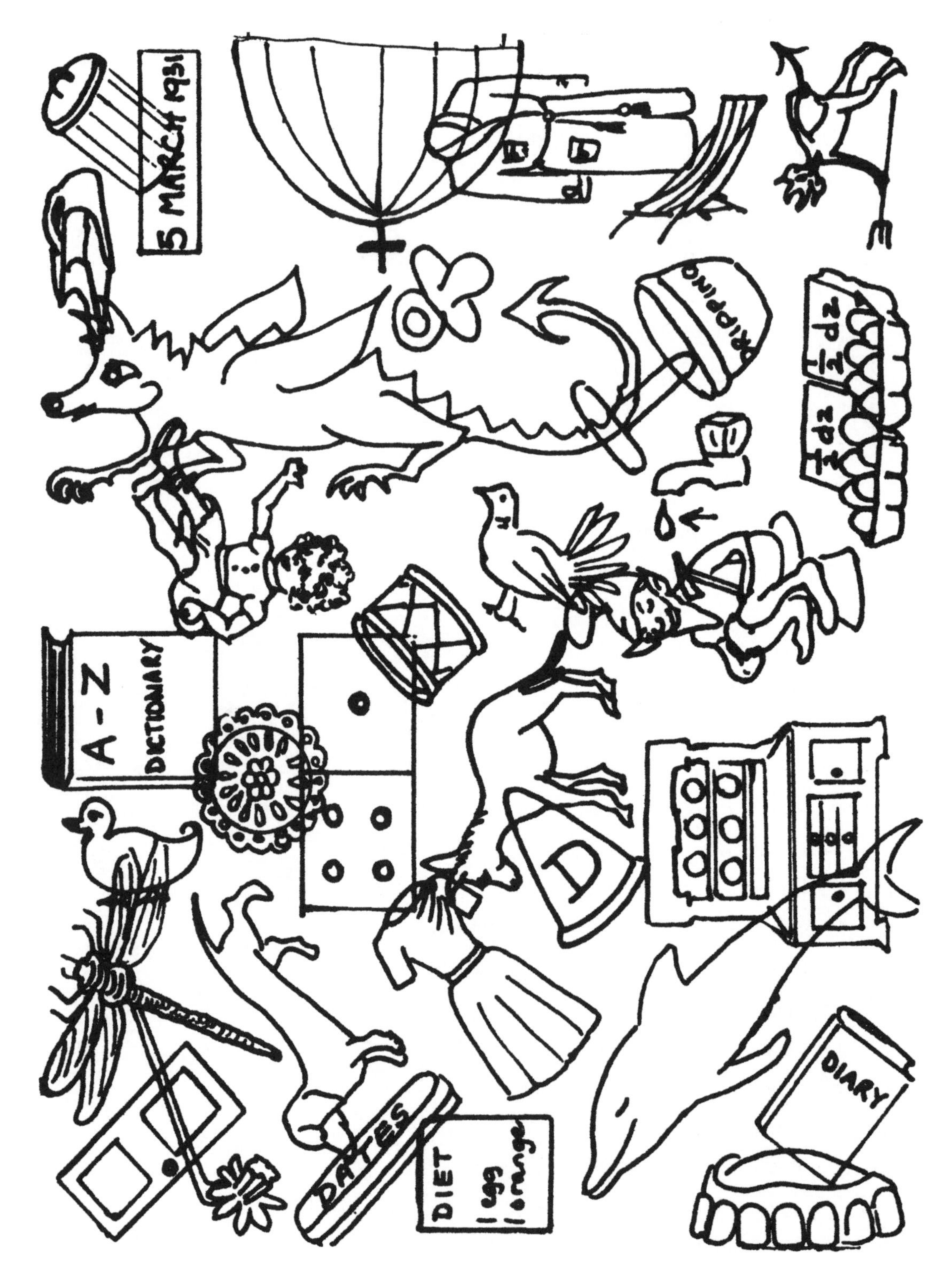

Answers: Deckchair, Date, Dome, Dibber, Dog, Dentures, Domino, Dictionary, Dustpan, Drum, Dove, Diet, Dustbin, Dragonfly, Dresser, Doily, Devil, Dragon, Donkey, Dolphin, Duck, Dates, Dozen, Doll, Door, Dunce's Cap, Dripping, Dressing Gown, Daffodil, Diary, Drop, Dress, Dwarf, Dummy

4. It's all Welsh to me

Write the following on the flipchart and ask the group to solve the sentences. The spaces between the words are not in the correct places. Can you put this right?

For example:
Th issent encei sno tqui ter ight. = This sentence is not quite right.

1. Pri nceCha rlesisthePr inceofWa les
2. Le eksi nche ese sau cea rego od
3. Ivo rtheE ngin eis onC hil dre n'sTV
4. Th eWe lshRu gby tea mise xcit ing
5. Swa nse aist hema inpo rtof Wal es
6. The rear eman ycas tlesi nWa les
7. Ang lese yisa lar geisla ndint heMe naistr aits
8. Thed affo dilis thef low ero fW al es

Answers

1. Prince Charles is the Prince of Wales
2. Leeks in cheese sauce are good
3. Ivor the Engine is on Children's TV
4. The Welsh Rugby team is exciting
5. Swansea is the main port of Wales
6. There are many castles in Wales
7. Anglesey is a large island in the Menai straits
8. The daffodil is the flower of Wales

5. Welsh quiz

(based on *Mental Aerobics* page 238)

Ask the group in general, or split into two teams called 'Leeks' and 'Daffodils'. If one team is unable to answer, pass question over to other team.

1. Who is Wales' greatest poet?...Dylan Thomas
2. Where was he born?...Swansea
3. What are cockles?...shellfish
4. What is laverbread made from?...seaweed
5. What is Wales' national game?...rugby
6. Where was the Prince of Wales' Investiture?...Caernarvon
7. Which English king was a Welshman?...Henry Tudor (Henry VII)

8. What language is Welsh derived from?...ancient Celtic
9. What channel separates Wales from England?...Bristol Channel
10. What is the highest Welsh mountain called?...Snowdon
11. What animal appears on the Welsh flag?...dragon
12. What is the Welsh national anthem?...'Land of my fathers'
13. What is the capital of Wales?...Cardiff
14. What are Welsh poets at the eisteddfods called?...Bards
15. The island separated by the Menai Straits from Wales?...Anglesey
16. Where most Welsh people worship...Chapel
17. Famous secondhand book fair...Hay-on-Wye
18. Name three industries of Wales...tourism, coal mining, steel, gold mining, slate mining
19. What is Dylan Thomas's most famous play?...'Under Milk Wood'
20. Famous Welsh actor who married Liz twice...Richard Burton
21. Famous Welsh actress who married Michael Douglas...Catherine Zeta Jones
22. Famous wild child with the voice of an angel...Charlotte Church
23. He sang many hymns and 'To the Snowman'...Aled Jones
24. He was a Goon...Harry Secombe
25. The longest place name in Wales?... LLANFAIRPWLLGWYNGYLLGOGERYCHWYRNDROBWLLLLANTYSILIOGOGOGOCH. (Can anyone say it?)
26. What does it mean, and where is it?...A small village on Anglesey famous only for its name! And it means: 'St Mary's church in the hollow of white hazel near a rapid whirlpool and the church of St Tysilio of the red cave.'

6. Singalong

Make list. How many Welsh songs can the group remember *and* sing?
Some suggestions:

- Wales, Wales, home sweet home is Wales
- We'll keep a welcome
- Land of my fathers
- Soss pan va (a rugby song)

When the Welsh songs run out, read out the following titles missing out the words in the square brackets. Ask for the missing word, and for the group to sing the song.

1. She's the [lily] of Laguna
2. Cruising down the [river]
3. I'm singing in the [rain]
4. I could have [danced] all night
5. The hills are alive with the [sound] of music
6. All things [bright] and beautiful
7. Where have all the [flowers] gone?
8. Run [rabbit] run
9. Three little [maids] from school
10. Love is the [greatest] thing
11. Daisy, Daisy give me your [answer] do
12. Land of [hope] and glory
13. There is a [tavern] in the town
14. Will you still [love] me when I'm 64?
15. I'll go no [more] a-roving
16. Climb every [mountain]
17. You are my [heart's] delight
18. Shine on [harvest] moon
19. Puff the [magic] dragon
20. The green [green] grass of home

7. See how many words can be found in: CAERNARVON CASTLE.

Week 2 – Houses and homes

Equipment: flipchart, paper, pens, estate agent details of various local dwellings, dice. Copies of the picture quiz on page 56.

1. Reminiscence and discussion

Ask the group in turn what kind of house they lived in when they were children. Who owned it? If rented, can they remember how much the rental was? Who was responsible for repairs? How many rooms for how many people? Did they have to share a bedroom? A bed? What did they call the various rooms – lounge, sitting room or parlour? kitchen or scullery? Did they have a pantry? What was kept in it?

Did they have indoor sanitation? A privy? Outside lavatory? Anyone ever seen an earth toilet? Did they have a bathroom? Was this upstairs or downstairs? If downstairs, was it put in later? Did they have piped water? What kind of heating did they have? (If solid fuel, who fetched sticks and coal? Who lit the fires?) On what type of stove did their mother cook? What kind of lighting did they have?

Did they live on an estate? Detached? Terraced? Back-to-back? Isolated farm/cottage? What was the house built from? Was it damp? What kind of flooring was in the house? Did they have carpets or lino? What was the roof like? What outbuildings did they have? A washhouse? Shed? Coalshed? Lavatory? Barn? Stables?

Where did they live when they first got married or left home? Did they have to live with in-laws? Did they buy or rent? How much? How did they furnish their homes? Did they save up for things or use hire purchase? Can they remember their first big buy? How did they feel when they finally owned it? (On the flipchart write the amounts paid for homes to compare with today's prices. Ask staff what they paid for their first homes, and write alongside to illustrate.)

Ask everyone where they live now – if in residential home, ask where they came from (if not too emotional).

Did they do the decorating, DIY, in their homes? Was it easy or a cause of conflict between partners? What was their biggest/funniest mistake? Do they like the makeover shows on TV? Would they have allowed *Changing Rooms* to do things to their homes?

2. Estate agents

Give everyone paper and pen, then pass round details of a house (first, block out the price) and ask everyone to write down what they think it is worth. Do this with five or six houses in various localities. Ask everyone to say what they have written as their estimate, then reveal the actual asking price. Inform the group of all the costs now incurred in buying a house...stamp duty, estate agent fee, solicitor's costs, removal firm, carpets and curtains. Discuss HIPs (Home Information Packs) – which make the sellers responsible for information packs about their homes. Talk about 'chains'. Say how nearly everyone will have to pay Inheritance Tax because of the huge increase in house prices. (If the Chancellor has raised the limit, inform the group of the limit now.) Many people 'downsize' to release capital from their houses. Has anyone done this? From what to what?

3. Who lives in–? quiz

Ask individuals in turn, or as a group:

den...fox

burrow...rabbit

holt...otter

kennel...dog

cage...bird

teepee...American Indian

cave...bat

convent...nun

hotel...guests

barge...bargee

hutch...rabbit
stable...horse
barn...cows
fold...sheep
igloo...Inuit/Eskimo
castle...king
shoe...old Woman
nest...bird/ant
eyrie...eagle
palace...the Queen
sty...pig
croft...farmer in Highlands
pen...pig
lair...wolf
sett...badger
hive...bees
caravan...gypsy
shanty...dispossessed poor
manse...minister
halls of residence...students
form...hare
harem...sultan's wives/concubines
vicarage...vicar
villa...holidaymaker/retired Brit
ranch...cowboy
shop doorway...vagrant
tent...scout/camper
hovel...poor people
mansion...rich/landed gentry
garret...artist
aviary...birds
dray...squirrel
lodge...beaver/lodge keeper
hacienda...mexican rancher

Add more of your own, or ask the group to do so.

4. Build-a-house 'Beetle'

In teams called 'Palaces' and 'Castles', or individually, at tables of four.
Draw a house by rolling the dice in turn. List the values on the flipchart.

1 = doorknob
2 = chimney
3 = front door
4 = window (will need four windows)
5 = a wall/base (will need two walls and a base, so three scores of 5)
6 = roof

5. DIY differences

Give everyone a copy of the carpenter puzzle on page 56 – there is one small difference in each picture compared to the others.

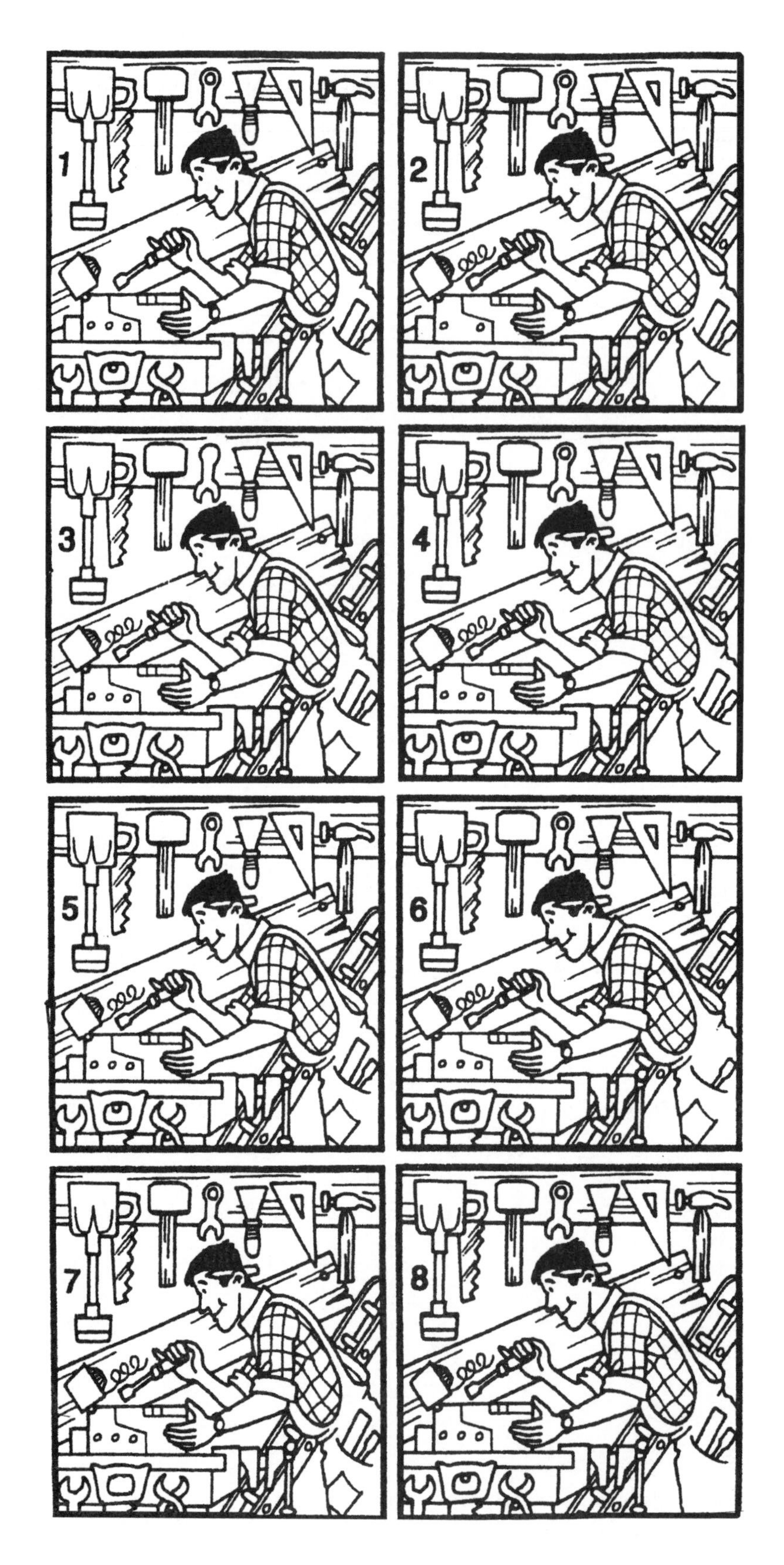

Answers: 1. wood shaving missing; 2. screw missing on vice; 3. no hole in spanner hanging up; 4. nail missing from end of plank; 5. no watch; 6. ruler missing from pocket; 7. no nail holding up saw on bench; 8. no patch on trouser leg

Week 3 – St Patrick's Day and Ireland

Equipment: flipchart, pens, paper, *River Dance* video, copies of word search on page 62.

1. Reminiscence and discussion

Ask the group if anyone has visited Ireland. How did they travel? Did they catch the ferry? Where from? What was their crossing like? Did they try Guinness? Did they like it? Is it true that it tastes better in Ireland? On the flipchart list all the things that remind the group of Ireland. Some prompts:

- Guinness
- leprechaun (an Irish fairy who is a shoemaker, he has a hidden pot of gold and is fierce in its defence, but if caught can be forced with threats of violence to reveal its hiding place – but if his captor takes his eyes off him, the leprechaun vanishes)
- Blarney Stone (a stone set in the wall of Blarney Castle – kissing it bestows the gift of eloquence on the kisser, i.e. the gift of the gab! You have to lie on your back and, holding onto a metal bar, bend backwards to reach the stone. This has been happening for over 500 years...imagine all those kisses – yuk!)
- Potato Famine (caused by blight damaging the staple crop and forcing many families to emigrate)
- IRA (all being well, now disbanded freedom fighters wanting an Ireland independent from the UK)
- Irish dancing (ask if the group would like to watch the 'River Dance' video)
- harp
- Orange Marches (also, we hope, now reduced in importance, where the Orange (Protestant) Order Apprentice Boys march around Belfast to commemorate the Battle of the Boyne and William of Orange)
- Emerald Isle
- Republican folksongs
- the Troubles and the sad history of Ireland
- links with Liverpool
- Irish Eyes
- Danny Boy
- horse racing
- navvies – gangs of itinerant labourers who travelled the country looking for work – they built the railways and canals in the nineteenth century
- paddies (a nickname derived from 'Patrick')
- luck of the Irish

- shamrock
- St Patrick
- St Bridget, another Irish patron saint.

Ask if anyone knows the legend of Saint Patrick. He was originally a Welsh priest who had a mission to convert the pagan Irish. He used the shamrock to illustrate the Holy Trinity and show how the Father, Son and Holy Ghost could exist as separate elements of the same entity. The day he died, 17 March 461 AD, became his saint's day and, though originally a Catholic holy day, is now celebrated worldwide as a more secular holiday. It was said that Patrick drove the snakes from Ireland (they were never native to Ireland). Some people think this was a metaphor for converting the pagans, as snakes were seen as pagan icons.

Can the group list any Irish songs...*and* sing them? 'When Irish eyes are smiling', 'Danny Boy', 'I'm looking over a four-leafed clover', 'My wild Irish rose', etc.

Read out these traditional Irish blessings:

May the road rise up to meet you,
May the wind be always at your back,
May the sun shine warm upon your face,
The rains fall soft upon your fields,
And until we meet again,
May God hold you in the palm of His hand.

May your blessings outnumber the shamrocks that grow,
And trouble avoid you wherever you go.

May you have the hindsight to know where you've been,
The foresight to know where you're going,
And the insight to know when you're going too far.

Does the group know any more?

2. How green am I?

(based on *Mental Aerobics* page 264.)

Ask the group in general.

1. I was found under a Royal mattress.
I am small and round.
I can be sweet.
pea

11. I am precious.
May is my especial month.
I have an Isle.
emerald

2. I have a wrinkled skin.
   Myth and legends are my haunts.
   I breathe fire.
   dragon

3. I live in water and on land.
   I could be in your throat!
   The French like my legs.
   frog

4. I grow in the sunny lands.
   I can be made into marmalade.
   I am from the citrus family.
   lime

5. I do not live in Ireland but many of my kind are green.
   I have no legs.
   I can poison or crush my prey.
   snake

6. I was stomped by feet.
   I turn 'white'.
   My cork is often 'screwed'!
   green grape

7. I grow on a tree.
   My oil is good for you.
   I decorate a pizza or Martini.
   olive

8. I have three parts.
   I am lucky.
   I am Irish.
   shamrock

9. I am round.
   I am always with red and amber.
   Vehicles move when I show.
   green traffic light

10. I am fodder.
    Children like to play on me, even when warned to 'keep off'.
    I need frequent cutting.
    grass

12. The forest is my home.
    I grow well in damp areas.
    I can have 'maidenhair'.
    fern

13. I'm good in salads and soup.
    I have white stalks.
    I have a heart.
    celery

14. I am also a fresh flavour.
    The first part of my name is a weapon.
    I flavour chewing gum.
    spearmint

15. I am part of Christmas.
    My leaves have prickles.
    My red berries feed the birds.
    holly

16. I am a small, wriggly eating machine!
    Gardeners dislike me.
    I become beautiful in the end.
    caterpillar

17. I am an after-dinner treat.
    I am a thick liquid.
    I have a French name.
    crème de menthe

18. I fly especially on this saint's day.
    I share space with orange and white.
    I am emblematic of Ireland.
    green stripe on the Irish flag

19. I am a well-known 'waiting' tune on the telephone.
    I was supposedly written by Henry VIII.
    Part of me is a from a gown.
    'Greensleeves'

20. I am warm and sheltering.
    I grow exotic plants.
    Small boys sometimes break my panes.
    greenhouse

Add more of your own.

3. 'IRE'-land words

(from *More Mental Aerobics* page 132.)

All the answers have 'IRE' in them. This could be a written, individual/group task, or written on the flipchart.

1. Sleepy…tIREd
2. On a police car or an ambulance…sIREn
3. Anger…IRE
4. Girl's name…IREne
5. Straight…dIREct
6. Dreadful…dIRE
7. Manager…dIREctor
8. Immediately…dIREctly
9. Combustion…fIRE
10. Warning of this…fIRE alarm
11. Gun…fIREarm
12. Heard on Bonfire Night…fIREworks
13. A glowing insect…fIREfly
14. Where you burn wood and coal…fIREplace
15. To employ someone…hIRE
16. Wet, soggy ground…mIRE
17. Blood sucker…vampIRE
18. To become known…transpIRE
19. Wearisome…tIREsome
20. Top of a church…spIRE
21. To die…expIRE
22. Fill with hope…inspIRE
23. Sweat…perspIRE
24. Is governed by an emperor…empIRE
25. Republic of Ireland…E-IRE
26. Cat in *Alice in Wonderland*… CheshIRE
27. Title of country gentleman…squIRE
28. Thin string of metal…wIRE
29. No longer at work/or gone to bed…retIREd
30. Churned-up mud…quagmIRE

Add more of your own.

4. Fairytale quiz

(based on *Mental Aerobics* page 26)

The Irish love the 'Little People', so play this in teams. One person from each team writes down the answers. Call the teams 'Leprechauns' and 'Shamrocks' and exchange answers for marking.

1. This wee man spun gold from straw…Rumpelstiltskin
2. She went to the ball…Cinderella
3. She pricked her finger and slept for 100 years…Sleeping Beauty

4. The Three Bears found her in their house...Goldilocks
5. Beware of her Grandma...Little Red Riding Hood
6. This clever cat made his master rich...Puss in Boots
7. The idle boy in this story sold a cow for magic beans...Jack and the Beanstalk
8. Her long hair saved her...Rapunzel
9. The shoemaker was secretly helped during the night...The Elves and the Shoemaker
10. They ate a house!...Hansel and Gretel
11. A wolf huffed and puffed...Three Little Pigs
12. She was so, so tiny...Thumbelina
13. A lovely girl who realised beauty is just skin deep...Beauty and the Beast
14. These children were saved by fairies and birds of the forest...Babes in the Wood
15. He never grew up, and lost his shadow...Peter Pan
16. Only one little boy was brave enough to tell the truth...The Emperor's New Clothes
17. Some little men, a talking mirror and a poisoned apple star in this tale...Snow White
18. A Genie in a magic lamp...Aladdin
19. 'Open Sesame' is the password...Ali Baba and the Forty Thieves
20. He was a famous rodent controller...The Pied Piper of Hamelin
21. The Troll under the bridge is in this story...Three Billy Goats Gruff
22. There is bronze statue of her to commemorate Hans Christian Andersen...The Little Mermaid

Ask the teams to set further clues for each other, or add more of your own.

5. Irish word search

Give everyone a copy of the grid on page 62.

6. See how many words can be found in this phrase, which means 'Ireland forever': ERIN GO BRAGH

7. Watch the 'River Dance' video, and maybe do a sitting-down jig!

L	E	P	R	E	C	H	A	U	N
A	G	O	F	Y	D	U	J	I	G
I	R	I	S	H	I	J	G	I	R
S	D	U	B	L	I	N	B	L	A
N	E	Y	S	T	R	I	S	H	J
I	R	E	L	A	N	D	S	T	P
A	R	A	I	N	B	O	W	B	L
S	H	A	M	R	O	C	K	A	N
G	O	O	D	L	U	C	K	E	L
T	O	B	L	A	R	N	E	Y	K

Can you find the following words? LEPRECHAUN, JIG, IRELAND, DUBLIN, IRISH, RAINBOW, SHAMROCK, GOOD LUCK, BLARNEY

Week 4 – The equinox, clocks and time

Equipment: flipchart, paper, pens, 'After Eight' chocolates, 'Your Stars' from various newspapers and magazines (to compare), signs of the Zodiac stuck on card without their names, playing cards

1. Reminiscence and discussion

Talk with the group about the clocks going forward this weekend – did they remember? Any funny stories about forgetting to change the clocks? Has anyone a way of remembering which way the clocks change? Here is one: *Spring forwards – Fall backward* (NB autumn is called 'fall' in USA.) Talk about the equinox – this is a Latin word which means 'equal night'. It now refers to either of the two times in the year when the sun crosses the plane of the Earth's equator and the day and night are of equal length. After the *spring equinox* the sun follows a higher and higher path through the sky, with the days growing longer and longer until it reaches the highest point in the sky on the *summer solstice.* It then starts to follow a lower path until it is at its lowest point at the *winter solstice.*

Who wound the clocks in the house when they were young? Did they have a grandfather, grandmother or granddaughter clock, or a cuckoo clock? Have they still got it? Can they describe it? Many of the old clocks incorporated the seasons and the waxing and waning of the moon. Could they see the pendulum? What sort of chime did their clocks have? Was it every quarter or on the hour? What was the tick like? Do they like to hear a clock ticking? Can they sleep with one ticking? How do they wake in the mornings? Alarm clock or radio alarm? What time do they rise?

Did anyone get a clock or gold watch when they retired? Have they still got it? Do they think this is a strange way of marking retirement? – especially as it is no longer important to be on time! Did they get a watch for their twenty-first or eighteenth birthday? How many clocks have they got?

Discuss the importance of ways of measuring time for mankind – so that we would know when to plan nomadic activity, when sacred feasts should be held, when to plant crops, how old we are, when we should do certain things.

Try an experiment: cover/hide the clocks and ask everyone to cover their watches, then ask everyone in turn what time they think it is. Keep a note, then see who is closest. Some people will be very accurate – often the ones who are very punctual and time-aware. Ask everyone how they feel about punctuality and how others' sense of time affects them. Talk about the different time zones in the world and how we cross them going on holiday, and suffer from jetlag.

Time was measured in the past with hourglasses, graduated candles, water clocks and sundials – perhaps the most ancient scientific instrument. Probably the first sundial was a pole in the ground with the length and direction of the shadow giving the time of the day. By the middle of the second millennium BC there were fixed and portable ones being manufactured. The height of the sun in the sky indicated the time by the length and direction of the shadow it produced. This was not very accurate, as the shadow varies at certain times of the day from season to season. In the twelfth century there were directional dials with the *gnomon* (the part of the dial that casts the shadow) set parallel to the Earth's axis. Does anyone have a sundial? What is its major drawback in the UK? (It needs sun!)

The hourglass was made up of two glass bulbs connected by a narrow neck. When turned upside-down, a measured amount of sand flowed through the neck in an hour. Can anyone say what the modern version of this is? (The egg timer.)

The water clock was an evenly marked container with a spout that allowed water to drip out at a given pace, and the time was indicated by the level the water in the container reached.

Pope Sylvester invented one of the earliest clocks in the tenth century. Now we have digital clocks and the time 'pips' on the BBC. Which clock chimes the hours on the media? (Big Ben) Is there a special chiming clock in the area nearby? Some towns have mechanical figures that strike the hour, has anyone seen one of these? Perhaps a visit could be arranged.

Ask the group about their concept of time. Have they noticed how time seems to pass very quickly when they are enjoying something and how it really drags when they are sad or waiting for something? Has time appeared to speed up as they got older? Can they recall that summer holidays seemed to stretch on forever when they were little?

What time do they awake? get up? Do they like an early cup of tea? What time do they go to bed? Do they wake in the night? Does the group like or dislike that strange time just between night and dawn? Any tips on getting back to sleep? Have they heard the dawn chorus?

Do they think their pets have a sense of time? Do they know when it is feeding time? Do they 'know' what time a family member is coming home? What is their favourite time of the day? Why?

Give everyone a 'taste of time' – an 'After Eight' mint!

2. A question of time – true or false?

See how the group answer these 'timely' questions – in teams – called 'Tick' and 'Tock'. Or answer individually. (Correct answers are in bold.)

1. On a digital clock you only see numbers for the hours, minutes and seconds of the current time. **True** – False
2. There are hands on a digital clock. **False** – True
3. A.M. stands for: **ante meridiem** – ante morning – ante midnight
4. P.M. stands for: post morning – **post meridiem** – post midnight
5. The a.m. time is from: noon till midnight – **midnight till noon** – midafternoon till midmorning
6. If it is 2pm on the 12-hour clock, what is it on the 24-hour clock? 13.00 **14.00** 22.00
7. The shortest hand on the clock measures: seconds – minutes – **hours**
8. How many minutes in an hour and seconds in a minute? 12 – 24 – **60**
9. How many minutes in two hours? 24 – **120** – 240
10. If it is 1:30, what time will it be in 45 minutes? 2:45 – **2:15** – 2:05

3. Sayings and songs

Ask the group to name and sing songs related to time. For example:

- Rock around the Clock
- Apple Blossom Time
- Hickory, Dickory, Dock
- As Time Goes By
- Unchained Melody
- My Three O'Clock Thrill
- My Grandfather's Clock
- Just in Time, I found you.

Add more of your own.
Gather some 'timely' sayings. For example:

- A stitch in time saves nine
- More haste, less speed
- Time and tide wait for no man
- Stands the clock at ten to three?
- News at Ten
- Procrastination is the thief of time.

Add more of your own.

4. Time zones

When it it 12 noon GMT in London, what time is it in these places?

1. New York
   5 hrs earlier
2. Sydney
   10 hrs later
3. Moscow
   3 hrs later
4. Mexico
   6 hrs earlier
5. Tokyo
   9 hrs later
6. Los Angeles
   8 hrs earlier
7. Seychelles
   4 hrs later
8. Samoa
   11 hrs earlier
9. Solomon Isles
   11 hrs later
10. Auckland
    12 hrs later
11. Sri Lanka
    5½ hrs later
12. Singapore
    8 hrs later

5. Group 'clock patience'

If you have large playing cards, use them as a group activity. If not, split into smaller groups and use ordinary packs. Deal all the cards out in clock formation, with four in the centre. Then take turns to turn a card and place it at the relevant clock place in the circle. When all Kings (placed in the centre) are turned over, re-shuffle and set out again.

6. See how many words can be made from: GREENWICH MEAN TIME.

Activities for April

Week 1 – Easter, a moveable feast

Switch the themed activities for March–April according to the date of Easter.

Equipment: flipchart, paper, pens, eggs, hardboiled or fresh, if allowed; collect 'blown' eggshells to decorate and hang on an Easter egg tree, little chocolate eggs for prizes, bits and pieces (ribbons, feathers, scraps of felt, buttons, costume jewellery, toy chickens, eggs, silk flowers) to make Easter bonnets out of old hats from charity shops or unwanted ones from staff, or invite people to bring in their own hats to decorate. Simnel cake to share.

1. Reminiscence and discussion

Talk with the group about the Easter celebrations they had when they were young. Did they have Easter eggs? Were they hardboiled eggs? How did they decorate them? Did they use vegetable dyes like onion skins? Did the group have chocolate eggs? Did their mothers make them or were they bought? Did they have to find them in the garden? Who hid them? Were they told the Easter Bunny hid them? Did they roll hardboiled eggs down a hill? Was there a special hill to do this? Was it a community affair? How was the winner decided – the person whose egg remained intact when it reached the bottom of the hill? Did they have egg-and-spoon races?

Do people buy Easter eggs now? What do they cost? Does the group feel they are too expensive for what they are? Is it all packaging? If they don't buy eggs for their grandchildren, do they buy something else?

Does the group know why we have eggs at Easter? Eggs are symbols of fertility and new life. The name of Easter comes from the name of the Anglo-Saxon goddess of the dawn, 'Eostre'. In pagan times there was a spring festival celebrated in her honour. They baked a special cake similar to our hot cross buns. When Christianity came to Britain this festival was incorporated in the celebration of the Resurrection of Jesus. Originally the eggs were painted in bright colours to represent the spring. Different countries have their own ways of egg decorating – the Greeks colour theirs crimson to represent the Blood of Christ, Germany and

Austria give green eggs on Maundy Thursday, while Slavic countries decorate theirs in gold and silver. Has anyone seen the fabulous Russian Fabergé eggs decorated with gold and jewels? They are goose or ostrich eggs and are carved with great precision, some even have hinged doors.

Did or does the group go to church at Easter? Did they get new clothes? Do they think we have lost the meaning of Easter? Is it too commercial? Before Easter comes do they send/receive Easter cards? Did they help their children make Easter bonnets for school? Have they been in a parade of Easter bonnets?

What is the special cake eaten at this time called? (Simnel cake, with marzipan balls to represent the Disciples.) Spring lamb is traditionally eaten on Easter Sunday.

2. Eggy crafts

Give everyone a hardboiled egg, or fresh if dyeing them. This activity is best with all sat around a large table with craft equipment in centre, but also works with a small central table with bits and pieces that the group requests from staff – this encourages participation and allows staff to assist easily. Some people may need encouraging to do this, as it could be a long time since they were involved with making things.

DECORATED EGGS

Tie leaves, ribbon or string around the fresh egg and boil it in water with onion skins or drops of food dye/cochineal in it. After about 8–10 minutes, allow to cool and take the string, leaves or ribbon off the eggs to reveal a pattern – all being well. Alternatively, decorate a hardboiled egg with crayon, pencil, felt-tipped pen, feathers, cardboard, etc. (At our Easter parties we always had a decorated egg competition and folk made wonderful specimens from Batman to Margaret Thatcher.) Display the eggs and get the group to vote for a winner. A small chocolate egg is the prize!

EASTER EGG TREE

During the week get people to save 'blown' eggs – when cooking, instead of breaking eggs, pierce both ends of the egg with a needle or small skewer and blow the contents into a bowl. (A reverse case of teaching your granny to suck eggs?) Give each group member an eggshell and ask them to decorate it *carefully* with felt tips or crayon. The eggs are then hung on the branches of a tree, which can be done by tying thread around half a matchstick (halved to fit inside shell). Push it downwards into shell, then ease until it is wedged across the hole, and tie onto a twig with the thread. When the wind blows it whistles through the shells, and when the sun shines the tree looks bright and festive.

3. Easter bonnets

Give everyone an opportunity to decorate a hat, then have a parade, take photos and invite a staff member to award first, second and third prizes, with a special prize for the men who dare!

4. Easter/springtime quiz

(based on *Mental Aerobics* page 273)

Ask the group in general.

1. When is the first day of Spring?...21 March
2. Name three spring flowers...Crocus, daffodil, hyacinth, narcissus, snowdrop
3. Who betrayed Jesus with a kiss?...Judas Iscariot
4. Handel wrote a famous oratorio for this time...*the Messiah*
5. What is the symbol of Christ's crucifixion?...The Cross
6. Which day celebrates Jesus' triumphal entry into Jerusalem?...Palm Sunday
7. Can you name the man who offered his tomb for the burial of Jesus?...Joseph of Arimathea
8. The 40 days of fasting before Easter are known as?...Lent
9. Jesus wore a crown of...thorns
10. How much did Judas betray Jesus for?...30 pieces of silver
11. The garden where Jesus was buried?...Gethsemane
12. The day before Lent begins is?...Ash Wednesday
13. The name of the hill outside Jerusalem where Jesus was crucified?...Golgotha (which means 'place of the skulls') or Calvary
14. Complete this springtime verse: 'March winds and April showers'...'Bring forth May flowers'
15. What is traditionally served with roast spring lamb?...mint sauce
16. Name two songs associated with springtime or Easter. Can you sing them?...'Tiptoe through the Tulips', 'April love', 'Easter Parade', 'April in Paris', 'I'll Be with You in Apple-blossom Time'
17. Who discovered the body of Jesus was missing from the tomb?...Mary Magdalene
18. What used to be done in most homes at this time?...spring-cleaning
19. What is the meal Jesus shared with the Disciples before His death known as?...the Last Supper
20. What did a young man's fancy do at this time?...'Lightly Turn to Thoughts of Love'.

5. Young at heart

Ask the group in general.
Name the young of the following:

frog...tadpole	goat...kid	man...child
cow...calf	rabbit...kitten	whale...calf
goose...gosling	pig...piglet	fish...fry

swan...cygnet	hen...chicken/chick	hare...leveret
sheep...lamb	duck...duckling	dog...puppy
horse...foal	lion...cub	cat...kitten

Ask the group for more examples.

6. Stones quiz

(from *Mental Aerobics* page 78)

There was a stone covering the mouth of the tomb where Jesus was buried. Can the group name these 'stone' words?

1. It represents each month of the year...birthstone
2. An imperial weight...stone (How many pounds in one? 14 pounds.)
3. A memorial...tombstone
4. Could be round your neck!...millstone
5. Sharpens knives...grindstone, whetstone
6. Helps you cross a stream...stepping stone
7. The main stone in an arch...keystone
8. Painful if you get one...kidney stone, gallstone
9. Make a pathway...flagstones
10. Count them to see who you'll marry...plum, cherry or peach stones
11. Imitation diamond, often on cowboy's clothes...rhinestone
12. Cartoon...'The Flintstones'
13. Game played on ice uses this stone...curling stone
14. A prime minister and a piece of luggage...Gladstone
15. Kiss this to talk a lot...Blarney Stone
16. A place of Druids...Stonehenge
17. Soft stone...sandstone
18. Famous US general...Stonewall Jackson
19. Wall without cement...drystone wall
20. Frozen raindrop...hailstone
21. Short distance away...a stone's throw
22. First stone of a building...cornerstone, foundation stone
23. Part of the fireplace...hearthstone.

7. A selection box

Chocolate anagrams. Write the anagrams on the flipchart for the group to solve individually.

KYRIALMT	Milk Tray
GBALMIKCCA	Black Magic
SROES	Roses
TQAUERETTYILS	Quality Street
YAXLAG	Galaxy
ELEONRTOB	Toblerone
HRRREFEORROEC	Ferrero Rocher
XDYAOIBR	Dairy Box
ORHEES	Heroes
TSROONNHT	Thorntons
BAMRASR	Mars Bar

8. See how many words can be made from: EASTER BONNET.

Week 2 – Spring-cleaning

Equipment: flipchart, paper, pens, quizzes, headscarves for the ladies. If you can find some old-fashioned cleaning equipment such as beeswax polish, feather dusters, carpet beater, carpet sweeper, old-fashioned mop and bucket, these always promote discussion. Copies of word search chart on page 72 and picture puzzles on pages 73, 74 and 76.

1. Reminiscence and discussion

Ask the group about the ways they used to cope with spring-cleaning – or avoid it, if they are male! When did they or their mothers or wives start to do it? Did they wear special clothes to clean in? Give the ladies a headscarf each and ask them to demonstrate how they wore it. Comment on different styles...are they regional?

Did they have a planned approach to their spring-cleaning? Where in the house did they start? Bottom floors up or bedrooms down? Did they have a specific method of cleaning a room? Remove and wash all ornaments? Shake rugs outside or through upper windows? Did they give or ask for assistance moving heavy furniture to clean underneath? Did anyone find anything interesting under things, such as previously lost items?

What did they use to clean carpets? Did they have a carpetsweeper? Can they remember the make? (Ewbank, possibly.) When did they get their first Hoover? What do they use now?

Any comments on today's big, heavy machines? Did people wash down paintwork and walls? Did they take down curtains, especially nets, and wash them, or change the winter ones for lighter summer ones? Was the winter bedding put away and cotton sheets substituted for flannelette? Where did they store the winter bedding?

How did they clean the windows? Did anyone hang out of their windows to clean them? Were they aware of risks? What did they stand on to reach things? What do they stand on now? (Good time to emphasise safety and fall prevention.) Any special cleaning tips? Anyone use old newspapers or vinegar and water to clean windows? How do they clean them today? Do they prefer to use a chamois leather? Did they recycle old clothes for dusters and cleaning cloths? What makes the best ones? Terry nappies were especially good – this could lead to a discussion on disposable versus washable nappies. Who cleaned or still cleans the silver/ brass in the house? What do they use? Did everyone have their own allotted household task when they were little?

Did the group use spring-cleaning to have a good clearout of old clothes and unused items? Where did they take them? Rag-and-bone man? What did he give them in exchange? How many people had a goldfish? How long did it live? Do they send things to charity shops today? Do they buy things in charity shops? Any good bargains? Do they line their clothing drawers? Does the group recycle waste? Do they know how it is used by councils? (NB often a representative from Environmental Health will come and give a talk about recycling, which is very informative.)

When they were young did their mothers have certain days when they did certain household tasks? Can they remember them? Monday, washing day – with cold meat and rice pudding for tea. Whatever the weather, washing was done. Tuesday, ironing; Wednesday, baking; Thursday, bedrooms; Friday, downstairs; and weekend, baking, etc. How was their week planned?

On the flipchart make a list of any household pests, where they could be found and how to deal with them – moths, silverfish, woodlice, house flies, spiders, mice, rats, carpet bugs, fleas from pets. Also make a list of any cleaning products the group can remember. Are they still available? (Vim, Chemco, Stardrops, Jiff, Zebra Black Leading, Ajax.) List any handy tips the group has – give some prompts. Ask the group first for their tip and if no one remembers any, write down the following to jog memories.

CLEANING TIPS

To remove:

- *Candle wax* – place a tissue /kitchen paper on the wax and rest a warm iron gently over it, keep replacing tissue as wax melts.
- *Chewing gum* – rub with an ice cube, and when it hardens gently scrape off with a blunt knife.
- *Magic marker pen* – spray with hairspray and gently wipe with soft cloth/kitchen roll.
- *Wine spill* – white wine: cover with table salt to soak up, then pat with damp cloth. Red wine: immediately cover with white wine, then use salt method above.

- *Blood* – soak in cold water, rub with cornstarch and dry in sun. Use diluted hydrogen peroxide if dried on.
- *Scratches from furniture* – shoe polish and felt-tipped pens will disguise small scratches. Water spots on furniture: allow to dry out completely, then rub with a little mayonnaise on a soft cloth.

To clean:

- *Chrome* – use soda water and a soft cloth.
- *Dirty collars* – rub cheap shampoo or Fairy Liquid into dirt before putting in washer.

2. Word search

P	M	D	U	S	T	P	A	N	A
F	E	A	T	H	E	R	M	O	P
F	K	X	H	R	E	T	S	U	D
C	M	O	T	H	B	A	L	L	S
H	L	E	A	T	H	E	R	P	B
A	Q	H	M	K	P	P	E	O	R
M	R	E	V	O	O	H	J	L	A
O	Z	Y	B	R	O	O	M	I	S
I	B	U	C	K	E	T	T	S	S
S	S	I	L	V	E	R	V	H	O

Can you find these hidden words?

FEATHER DUSTER, DUSTPAN, MOP, BUCKET, CHAMOIS LEATHER, SILVER POLISH, BRASSO, BROOM, MOTHBALLS, HOOVER

3. Spot the differences in these untidy rooms

Give everyone a copy.

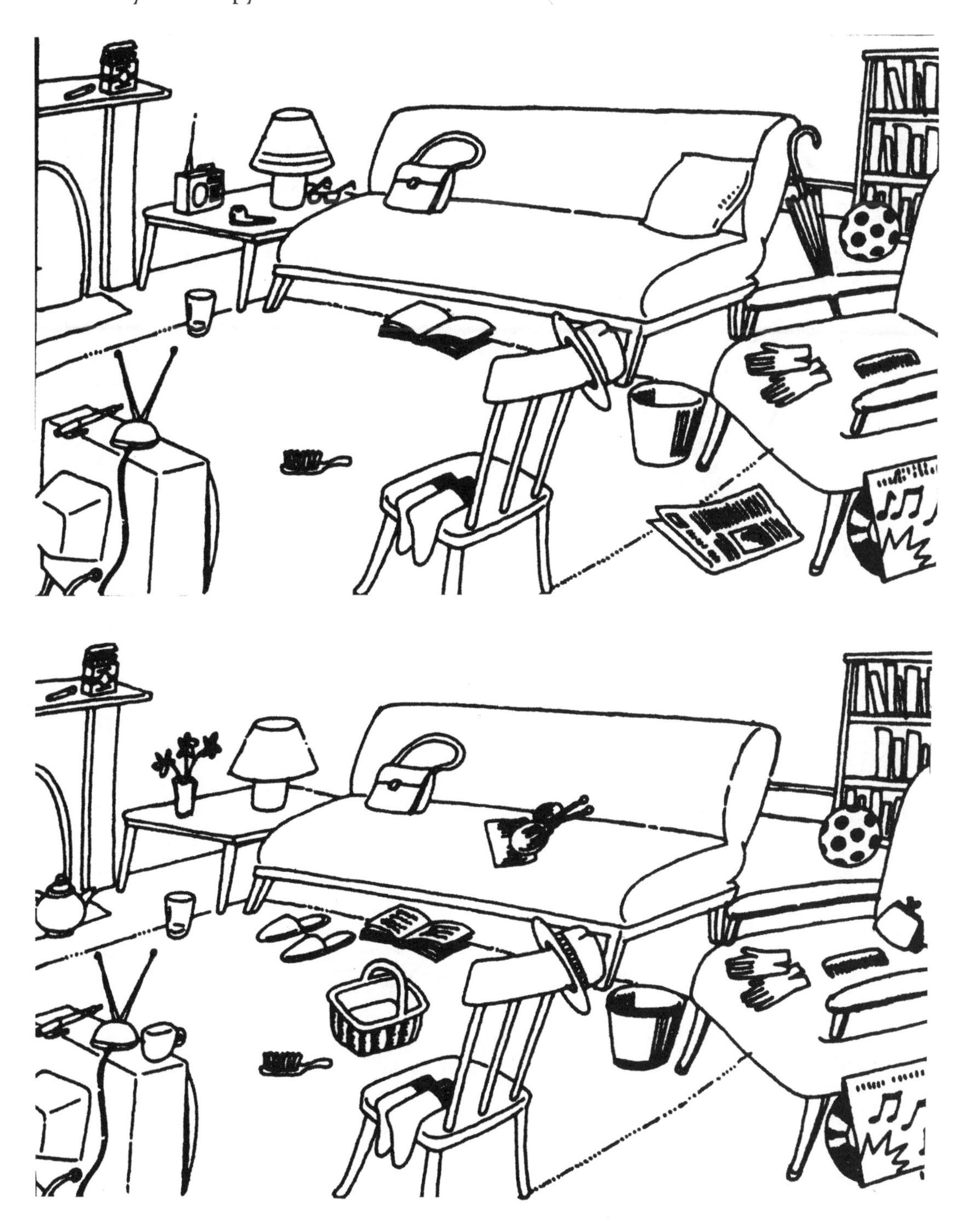

Answers: In top picture – cup missing from top of TV, teapot missing from hearth, radio in place of flowers on coffee table, table lampshade has stripes, glasses and pipe on table, no slippers under sofa, no writing in book, cushion on sofa but no knitting, umbrella missing, books missing, no purse on chair, waste bin missing stripes, newspaper under chair, extra musical note on record cover, hat on chair different, no basket on floor

4. A drawer to tidy

Give everyone a copy.
Can you list the different items? There are 26 of them!

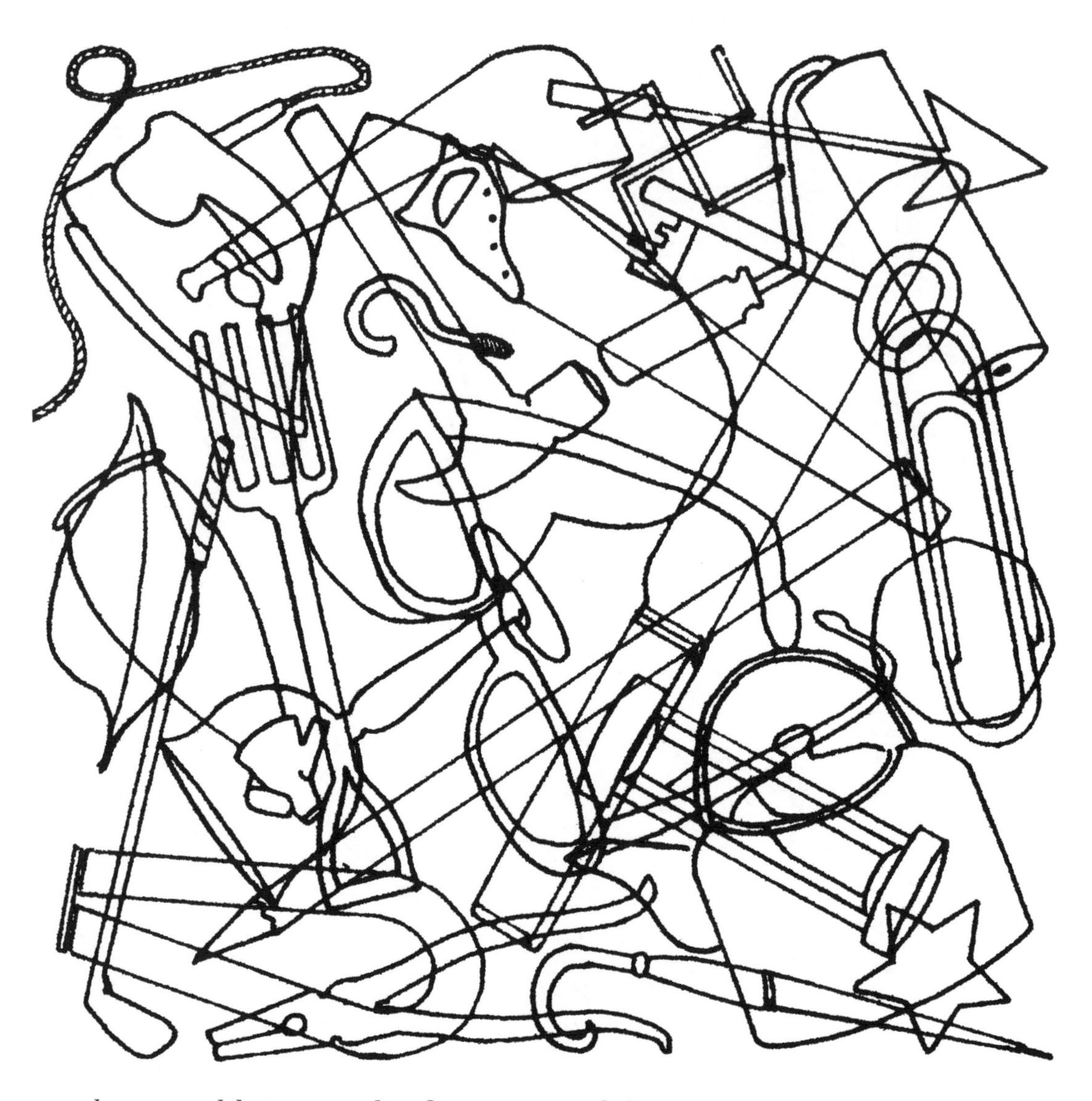

Answers: Key, saw, pipe, iron, leaf, star, hook, knife, heart, arrow, pliers, kettle, hammer, pencil, specs, umbrella, magnet, golf club, egg timer, swastika, paper clip, garden fork, wine glass, paint roller, 50p piece, soda siphon

5. House quiz

(from *Mental Aerobics* page 52)

Some more 'houses' to clean! Ask the group in turn.

1. Where the President of America lives…the White House
2. A house with lots of cash!…counting house
3. Where you go for your meal in the army…cookhouse

4. Just inside the grounds of a mansion...gatehouse
5. Not for commoners!...House of Lords
6. Book by Edgar Allan Poe...*The Fall of the House of Usher*
7. Famous women's magazine...*Good Housekeeping*
8. Where nautical craft are kept...boathouse
9. Where cowboys sleep at the ranch...bunkhouse
10. Classical singing takes place here...opera house
11. A den we climbed to...tree house
12. Tender plants are grown here...greenhouse
13. Home of Government...The Houses of Parliament
14. Where actors perform...playhouse
15. For storage of goods...warehouse
16. For canines or men in trouble!...doghouse
17. The very uppermost posh flat...penthouse
18. Where kippers are done to a turn...smokehouse
19. A dreaded place where the poverty-stricken were sent...workhouse
20. This has miniature furniture...dolls' house
21. In nursery rhymes...'The House that Jack Built', 'The Crooked House', 'A big shoe'!

6. Spring-cleaned rooms

How many differences can you find in the rooms on page 76?

7. See how many words can be found in: ELBOW GREASE.

Week 3 – Birds

Equipment: flipchart, pens, paper. Collect pictures of birds, laminate them if possible, to use as an identification quiz. OHP slide or copies of 'Name that bird' on page 78, copies of 'Bird search' on page 80.

1. Reminiscence and discussion

Ask the group if they ever kept birds? A budgie, parrot, canary? What did they call their bird? Could it 'speak'? What colour was it? How long did they have it? Do they still have a cage bird? Did anyone keep racing pigeons? Where were they kept? Any stories about their pigeons? Can they explain how they found their way home? (Pigeons mate for life and so, when separated, fly straight back to their mate.) Did they win any cups/prizes?

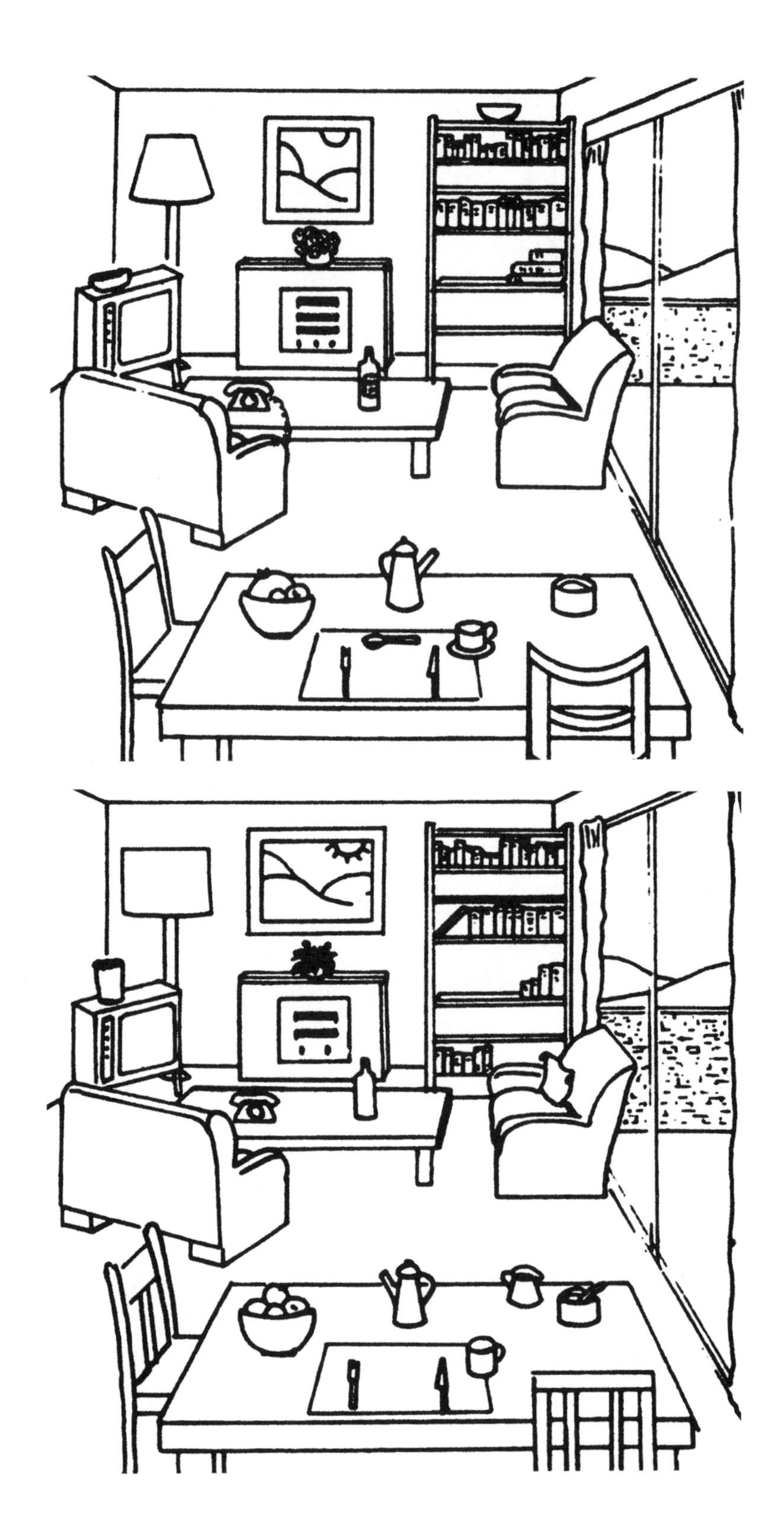

Answers: In bottom picture – chair backs different, saucer and spoon missing, milk jug and sugar spoon added, coffee pot facing different way, fruit in bowl different, no flex on phone, no label on bottle, different vase on TV, lampshade different, picture bigger and sun has rays, different flowers on fire, bar missing from fire, no bowl on book case, books different on 2nd and 3rd shelves and added to bottom shelf, cushion on sofa, pelmet missing, wall in garden bigger

Did anyone keep hens in their back garden or field? Who looked after them? What did they feed them on? Were they good layers? Did they actually eat them, or did they become too friendly with them to do this?

Does the group feed the birds? With what? Any stories about the stealing habits of the grey squirrel? What does the group feel about the proposed culling of the greys to help the reds survive? Does anyone have a birdtable? Birdbath? What birds have visited them? Does anyone have a nestbox in their garden? Is it used? Has anyone a story about finding a nest in an unusual place? (Robins often nest in sheds, even boots stored in sheds.) Did the house martins nest on their house? Did they know the old country saying that they only nest on happy homes? When they were young, did they go birdnesting? This is illegal nowadays, but often in the past boys collected eggs. Can they identify birds from their eggs? Has everyone seen a nest in the wild? Talk about the skills a bird has to actually build a nest. Ask about the types of materials that can be used – hair, sheep's wool, ferns, twigs, even mud and spittle.

Anyone have a story about a bird? One coming down a chimney? Flying into the house? Stealing shiny items? (Thieving magpie.) Tame jackdaw? Talking mynah bird causing trouble? Swearing parrot? Messing washing? Why is a bird messing on you lucky? It's always a third party who says this, I suppose because they are relieved it didn't hit them!

2. Bird songs

On the flipchart list how many songs/poems the group can think of connected with birds.

Suggestions

- Red, Red Robin
- A Nightingale Sang in Berkeley Square
- Bye, Bye Blackbird
- Chick, Chick, Chick, Chicken
- There Once was an Ugly Duckling
- Bluebirds over the White Cliffs of Dover
- Sing a Song of Sixpence
- Who Killed Cock Robin?
- Goosey, Goosey Gander
- O for the Wings of a Dove
- The Owl and the Pussy Cat
- Two Little Dickie Birds (Sitting on a Wall, One called Peter, One called Paul)
- The Thieving Magpie
- Poem: From out the Distant Forest an Owl Called out 'I'm Here' (Girl Guides will know this and may be encouraged to sing it)
- Morning has Broken.

3. Name that bird

Give everyone a copy or use an OHP if available.

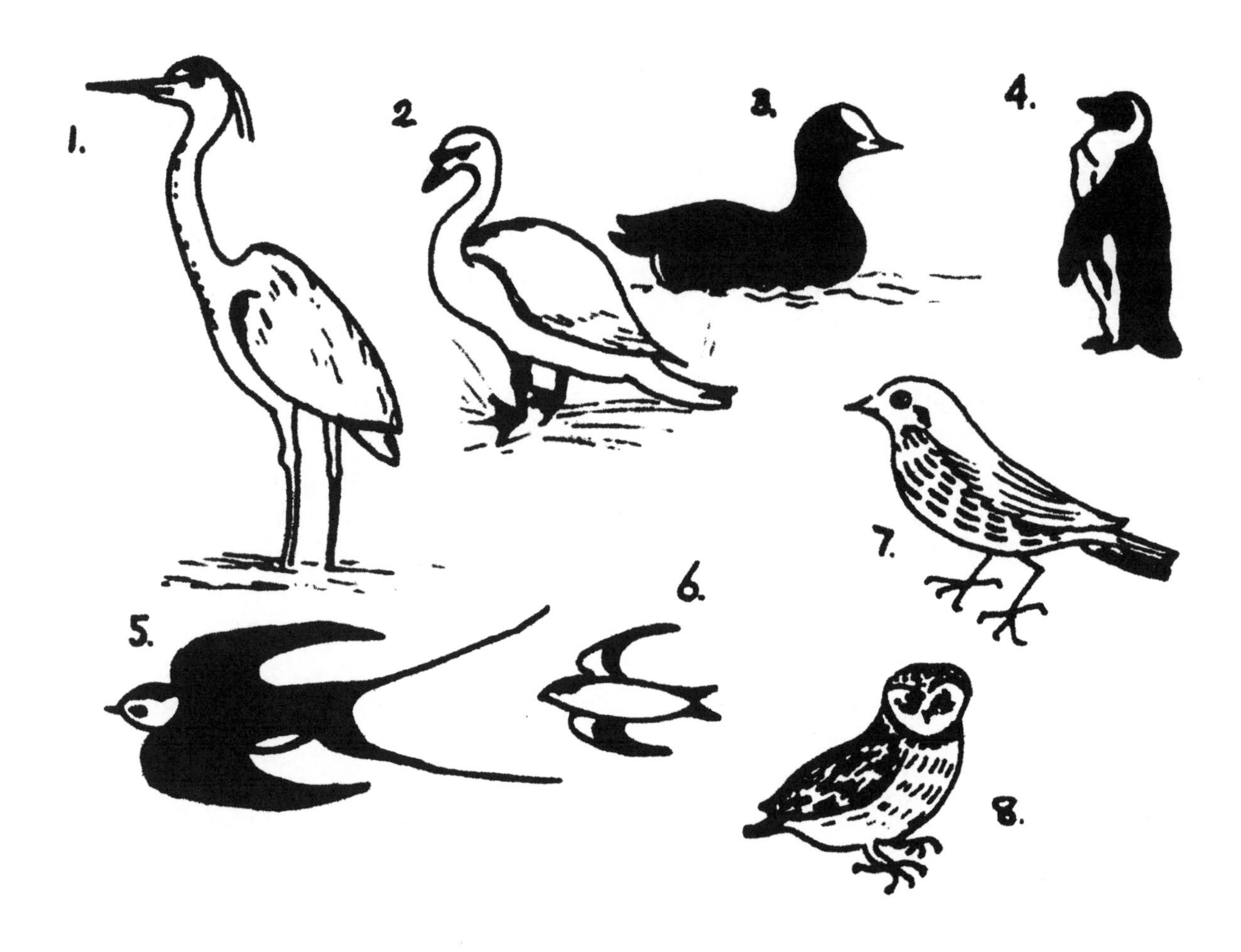

Answers 1. Heron, 2. Swan, 3. Coot, 4. Penguin, 5. Swallow, 6. House martin, 7. Thrush, 8. Owl.

4. Bird words

(from *More Mental Aerobics* page 107)

Ask the group in turn.

1. A royal angler…kingfisher
2. Bye, bye…blackbird
3. Brings babies…stork
4. Around the Ancient Mariner's neck…albatross
5. Proud fellow…peacock
6. Part of eating…swallow

13. He is short of breath…puffin
14. An ocean cons you…seagull
15. Jenny…wren
16. Little Red…hen
17. Symbol of Peace…dove
18. Woody…woodpecker

7. Does he not know the words?...hummingbird
8. Wise old...owl
9. Stool...pigeon
10. Batman's sidekick...robin
11. – clock...cuckoo
12. Dislikes Christmas...turkey
19. Florence...nightingale
20. A sitting...duck
21. Seen at the docks...crane
22. A precious bird...goldcrest
23. Hides his head in the sand...ostrich.

5. Hidden birds

Write these on the flipchart and ask the group to find them. Add more of your own.

NERAV	raven	OUESRG	grouse
RDIBKACLB	blackbird	NYRAAC	canary
WOLLWAS	swallow	KEPCACO	peacock
CHNICFFAH	chaffinch	ORCNOD	condor
NIRBO	robin	THESMANOUIR	house martin
AWSN	swan	KOOCUC	cuckoo
CHBLLUFNI	bullfinch	RUTHSH	thrush
ELEGA	eagle	NREW	wren
CHORIST	ostrich	WIFST	swift
EIPMGA	magpie	LITTACO	coal tit
LOW	owl	RHONE	heron
SSROTAABL	albatross	RULETUV	vulture
TOOKAOCC	cockatoo	STEGDROCL	goldcrest
TPNASHAE	pheasant		

6. Bird search

A case of ten birds in the hand and one in the bush?

R	A	V	E	N	B	C	V	E	D
B	B	L	A	C	K	B	I	R	D
C	H	A	F	F	I	N	C	H	B
L	K	N	R	O	B	I	N	H	U
S	W	A	N	M	T	J	E	J	D
N	P	K	E	A	G	L	E	F	U
M	O	S	T	R	I	C	H	S	C
C	O	N	D	O	R	H	D	R	K
S	I	S	W	A	L	L	O	W	S
B	L	U	E	T	I	T	S	X	H

Can you find the following birds?

RAVEN, BLUE TIT, CONDOR, OSTRICH, CHAFFINCH, ROBIN, EAGLE, BLACKBIRD, SWALLOW, SWAN, DUCK

7. Bird brain quiz

Ask the group in turn.

1. What my true love sent…a partridge in a pear tree
2. Messenger birds…pigeons
3. One is unlucky…magpie
4. The first one hears makes the news!…cuckoo

5. When birds fly away south, they...migrate
6. A bit of a card? Especially at Christmas...robin
7. Bringer of babies...stork
8. Their feathers warm us...eider duck
9. Alarming bird...cockerel
10. His beak can hold more than his belly can!...pelican
11. Which bird first left the Ark?...raven
12. Wise old thing...owl
13. The 'laughing' Australian bird...kookaburra
14. King of the birds...golden eagle
15. New Zealand rugby player...kiwi
16. He swims but doesn't fly...penguin
17. What colour is a female blackbird?...brown
18. It is very bad luck for the Crown if they leave the Tower...ravens
19. He became extinct in seventeenth century...dodo
20. He is known in the country as a yaffle and hammers on trees...woodpecker
21. Protected by the Queen...swans
22. Said to rise from the ashes...phoenix
23. This type of crow is pink and blue...jay
24. This range of books was the younger version of the Penguin...puffin.

8. See how many words can be made from: BIRD'S NEST SOUP.

Week 4 – St George's Day and England

Equipment: flipchart, pens, paper, red, white and blue jelly beans, St George's flags for decoration. Collection of red, white and blue items for Kim's Game. Copies of the picture quiz 'Sightseeing in London' on page 83.

1. Reminiscence and discussion

Ask the group if they know anything about St George. He was not an Englishman – probably never even visited these shores. He is thought to have been born in Turkey, around 1700 years ago, of Christian parents. On the death of his father he went with his mother to Palestine to manage her estates. There he joined the Roman army and rose to the rank of tribune (equivalent to a major today). His emperor was the cruel Diocletian, who persecuted the Christians without mercy. George was horrified at the treatment of his fellow Christians and went to plead their cause with the Emperor, but he was imprisoned and tortured. When he refused to denounce his religion he was dragged through the streets and beheaded. The wife of the Emperor was so impressed by his bravery that she converted to Christianity and was condemned to death.

After the Emperor Diocletian stepped down (one of the few emperors who did so) the cult of St George flourished. The oldest inscription of his name is dated 346 AD in a church in Syria. The Church of St George in Rome dates from the fourth century, and he was popular as a warrior saint in England in the 700s. Richard the Lionheart adopted him as his personal saint and his symbol of a red cross on white background became the flag of England. He became our patron saint in the fourteenth century. Edward III dedicated the Order of the Garter to him and the special chapel at Windsor Castle was created. The badge of the Order shows him slaying the dragon at Selene. (This could have been Libya or Cyrene, the Greek Christian stronghold.) Shakespeare famously had Henry V shout before the Battle of Agincourt in 1415, 'Cry God for Harry, England and St George!' In 1963 the Roman Catholic Church demoted George to a third-class saint, claiming there was little evidence he even existed, but in 2000 he was officially recognised as England's patron saint by Pope John Paul II. St George is also the patron saint of Moscow and Georgia and Aragon in Spain.

On the flipchart write the things the group feels define the English...their traits – stiff upper lip, fair play, being reserved, queuing, etc...their traditions – cricket on the village green, beefeaters, roast beef, royalty, castles, palaces, Tower of London, Chelsea Pensioners, morris dancers, warm beer, brass bands, crumpets, 'is there honey still for tea?' cups of tea, muffins, scenery, trains, great universities, Mother of Parliaments, etc... Ask the group in turn, 'Where is the best place in England that everyone should visit?'

Can the group name, and hum, any songs with 'England' in them? 'There'll always be an England', 'Who do you think you are kidding, Mr Hitler?', 'Mad dogs and Englishmen go out in the Midday Sun', even football songs will do.

2. Red, white and blue Kim's game

On a tray have a collection of red, white and blue objects (not too many). Show them to the group for two to three minutes, then cover them with a cloth and ask the group in turn what was red, then blue, then white... Keep a note of answers, then reveal tray once more. Those who guessed correctly can have a red, white or blue jelly bean.

3. Sightseeing in London

Give everyone a copy of the picture puzzle on page 83. Find the four sightseeing friends who are in all four pictures.

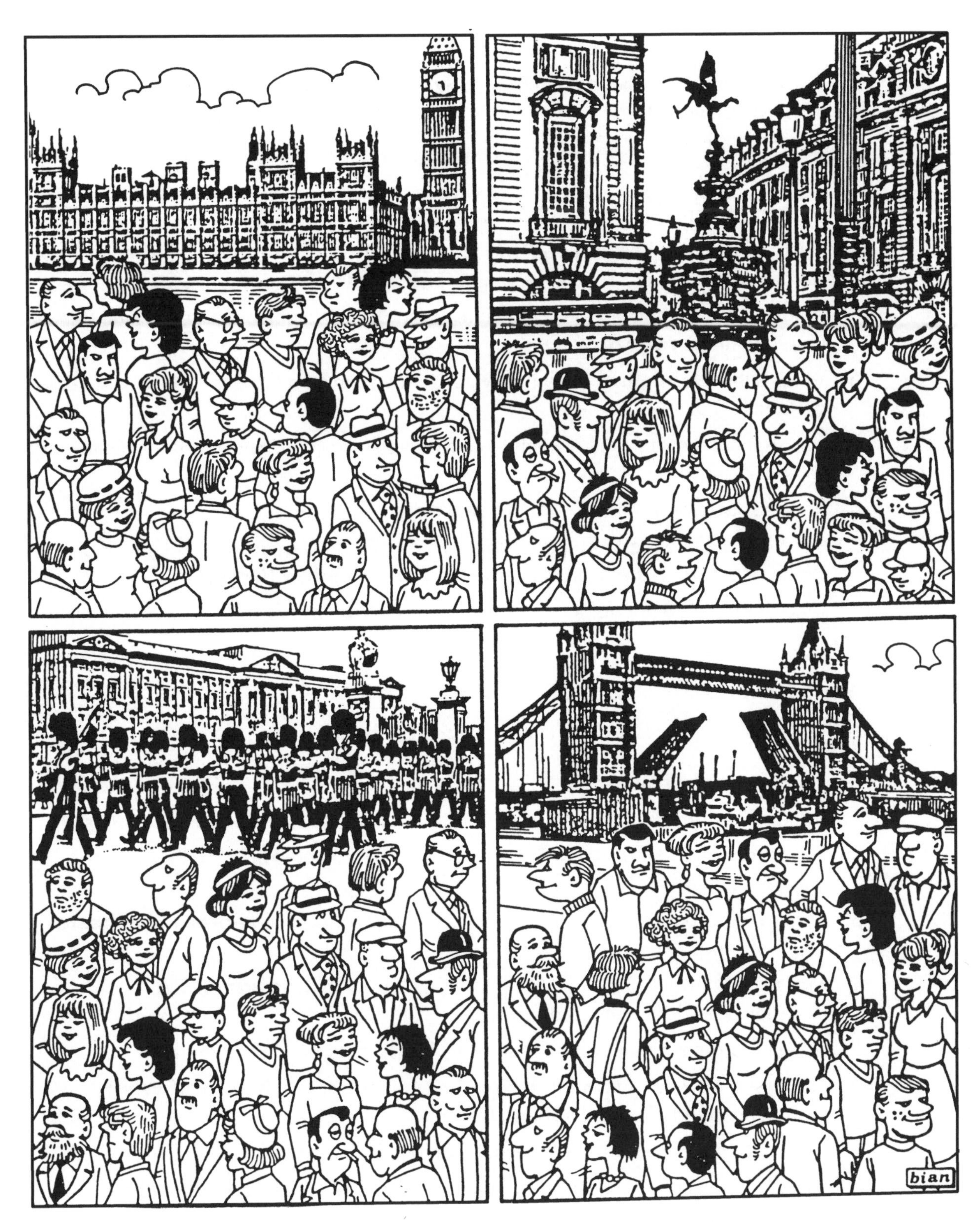

Answers: Woman with longish black hair, man in trilby with spotted tie, woman with short fair hair and earrings, man with black hair smoking a cigarette

4. Know your England

Ask the group to write down the initial letter of answers 1–9, so as to compose the answer to Question 10. (Correct answers are in bold type.)

1. The head of the Anglican church is the Archbishop of...**Canterbury**, York, Westminster or Oxford?
2. Which Suffolk town has a music festival?...Felixstowe, Sizewell, Ipswich or **Aldeburgh**?
3. Which river runs through Liverpool?...**Mersey**
4. Which library was built in 1662 and named for its founder?...British Museum Library, John Rylands, Radcliffe Camera or **Bodleian**?
5. What sporting events are held at Henley and Cowes?...horseracing, jousting, tennis tournaments or **regattas**?
6. What is the river Thames known as when it flows through Oxford?...**Isis**, Ox, Lethe or Avon?
7. The shortest sea route is between Calais and...Folkestone, Portsmouth, Felixstowe or **Dover**?
8. Kent is known as the – of England...**garden**
9. The botanical wonderland made from two Cornish clay quarries is called...Plant World, Plant Land, the Biosphere Experience or the **Eden Project**?
10. One of Britain's world famous university cities...**Cambridge**

5. Know your counties

Ask the group in general. Correct answers are in bold type.

These towns are in which county?

1. Totnes, Tiverton, Paignton, Newton Abbot...Dorset, **Devon**, Cornwall, Hampshire
2. Great Yarmouth, King's Lynn, Fakenham, Cromer...**Norfolk**, Cambridgeshire, Suffolk, Lincoln
3. Burnley, Blackburn, Preston, Blackpool...Greater London, **Greater Manchester**, West Midlands, Cumbria
4. Mansfield, Newark, Sutton in Ashfield, Worksop...**Nottinghamshire**, Leicestershire, Derbyshire, Staffordshire
5. Dover, Margate, Sittingbourne, Ashford...**Kent**, Essex, Wiltshire, Suffolk
6. Newcastle-on-Tyne, Sunderland, Gateshead, Tynemouth...**Tyne and Wear**, Northumberland, County Durham, Cumbria
7. Falmouth, Bude, Helston, Penzance...**Cornwall**, Dorset, Somerset, Devon
8. Stroud, Cirencester, Cheltenham, Tetbury...Warwickshire, **Gloucestershire**, Worcestershire, Herefordshire

9. Skegness, Boston, Sleaford, Grantham...**Lincolnshire**, Nottinghamshire, Cambridgeshire, Oxfordshire
10. Southport, Liverpool, Birkenhead, St Helens...**Merseyside**, Shropshire, Cheshire, Clywd
11. Dudley, Solihull, West Bromwich, Walsall...Staffordshire, **West Midlands**, Leicestershire, Warwickshire
12. Salisbury, Chippenham, Swindon, Devizes...Berkshire, Oxfordshire, Buckinghamshire, **Wiltshire**
13. Bury, Stockport, Oldham, Salford...Greater London, **Greater Manchester**, West Midlands, Cumbria
14. Poole, Bournemouth, Weymouth, Swanage...Kent, **Dorset**, Somerset, Hampshire
15. Basildon, Chigwell, Colchester, Braintree...Hertfordshire, **Essex**, Bedfordshire, Surrey

6. Saint George

On the flipchart write the following list:

- Girl's name
- Boy's name
- Town
- Country
- Flower
- Fruit
- Vegetable
- Animal
- Bird
- Job
- Hobby

Then, taking in sequence each letter of 'Saint George', ask the group in turn to give answers that begin with that letter, for example: *girl's name* – Susan, *boy's name* – Stanley, *town* – Stockport... Write the answers on the flipchart. If a letter is repeated (i.e. G or E), the answers must be different each time, if possible.

7. Where are these tourist spots?

Ask the group if they have been there?

1. Seaside town of lights...Blackpool
2. Where the Crown Jewels are kept...Tower of London

3. Home of the PM...10 Downing Street
4. England's monument to a famous naval commander...Nelson's Column
5. The Southwest corner of England...Land's End
6. Home of the tailless cat...Isle of Man
7. England's two most intellectual cities...Oxford and Cambridge
8. A London bridge that opens for the tall ships...Tower Bridge
9. London meat market...Smithfield
10. Where Shakespeare lived...Stratford-upon-Avon
11. Prehistoric monument near Salisbury...Stonehenge
12. A Roman wall to keep out the Scots...Hadrian's Wall
13. Home of the Beatles...Liverpool
14. A city with Shambles, a railway museum and the Jorvik Museum...York
15. The statue of Eros...Piccadilly Circus
16. The Norfolk waterway...the Broads
17. The Leeds Test Cricket Ground...Headingley
18. The Clifton Suspension Bridge...Bristol
19. Poet's Corner...Westminster Abbey
20. A theatre in Sheffield, home of televised snooker...The Crucible
21. The Photographic Museum...Bradford
22. Roman baths and the Crescent...Bath
23. The Ship Canal, built on the cotton trade, famously United...Manchester

Add more of your own.

8. Ask the group in turn to name their

a) Knight in shining armour (if a lady) – who they would most like to be rescued by.

b) Damsel in distress (if a gentleman) – who they would most like to rescue.

As a group who do they nominate as their Dragon?

Activities for May

Week 1 – May Day celebrations

Come all ye lads and lasses,
Join in the festive scene,
Come dance around the maypole
That will stand upon the green.

Equipment: flipchart, paper, pens, maypole, if possible – the cardboard inner tube of a carpet can be festooned with ribbons and flowers to make a decorative pole (make sure it is secure). And an invitation to the local morris men to perform! Copies of picture quiz on page 90.

1. Reminiscence and discussion

Talk about May Day celebrations in the past, did the group take part? Was one of them ever a May Queen? Was a May Queen part of the celebrations in their part of the country? Did they have new clothes for the May Day Marches? Did they pick wildflowers when they were young? This is not allowed now. Can they remember gathering arms full of bluebells? And being told off for bringing May blossom into the house? What is May blossom? Hawthorn, which blossoms at the beginning of May. Did they make daisy chains?

The traditions of May Day go back many centuries, as it is the celebration of the first day of summer, when the cattle were taken back out to pasture. It is the time for courtship and attraction – 'spring fever' – a time of flowers, fruits and dancing, especially around the maypole. It was widely believed that a damsel should wash her face in May Day dew to increase her beauty. People would get up at daybreak to gather flowers and blossoms to decorate the maypole, then, accompanied by a piper, they danced and sang around the pole – which was often seen as a fertility symbol.

Does anyone remember singing 'Here we come gathering nuts in May, On a cold and frosty morning'? The 'nuts' in this song are a corruption of the word 'knots' meaning bunches or nosegays of spring flowers – there are no nuts to gather in May. Can anyone sing it still?

Morris dancers often performed with their bells, ribbons and clashing sticks. The fairest girl was chosen as Queen for the day – sometimes a lad was chosen as King, and they led the village in the dances. There was often a Lord of Misrule selected, or even a Green Man (disguised in a cage of greenery – in fact, this still occurs in Castleton, Derbyshire, where a mounted man rides around the village covered by a wicker cage festooned with greenery and flowers). The couple could also be known as Robin Hood and Maid Marian, or even John Thomas and Lady Grey (shades of *Lady Chatterley's Lover*?). The festivities became so gay and abandoned, with the priest and nobility being the butt of many jokes, that the Puritans had them banned by Parliament – but as you can't keep a good celebration down, they soon emerged again and are still part of the life of many villages. Some northern areas have a celebration akin to April Fools' Day called May Gosling, when, if they trick anyone, they can call them a 'May Gosling', but after noon the tricked one can say 'May Gosling's past and gone, You're the fool for making me one.' In Padstow this is known as the 'Obby 'Oss Celebration, where they parade two giant hobby horses and the town is covered in bluebells and spring flowers.

Bluebells are a very potent flower associated with powerful magic, and at one time they were the symbol of Britain, before the Tudor Rose. Other names by which bluebells have been known are calver keys or culver keys (meaning the flowers resemble a bunch of keys), auld man's bell, Ring o' Bells, wood bells, jacinth, wild hyacinth. They are ancient plants and grow in ancient woodlands (we have a third of the world's bluebells in the British Isles), and much folklore is tied up with them. If you tread on a bluebell, the fairies will have you 'pixie-led' – led through the wood, unable to escape until someone rescues you. If you destroy bluebells near an oak tree, the oak tree fairies will take revenge on your pigs or your children. It is said the bluebell is a 'succubus' attractor. A succubus is an evil spirit that invades the bedrooms of men in order to procure a demon child, so men would put a bunch of bluebells in their room for protection, as it would attract the succubus away from them. Witches were said to grow bluebells to attract fairies to exchange magic spells with them…as ever, this was used against those poor old women accused of witchcraft, so any bluebells that happened to grow in their gardens were more or less a death sentence.

Monks used the bluebell to treat leprosy. In Wales it was used as a treatment for TB – as often with old wives' tales, research has found them high in alkaloids, which are effective against antibiotic-resistant TB.

The tradesmen and guilds celebrated their patron saints and entered floats in the May Day parades. The guilds were predecessors of trade unions. The shoemakers' saint is St Crispin, and for fairly obvious reasons the Guild of Tailors has Adam and Eve for theirs. There is a Sweep's Festival in Rochester, when the chimneysweeps traditionally downed brushes to have some fun.

May Day has become more and more a working class holiday, and we now have two May Bank Holidays, with 1 May being a celebration of workers everywhere.

2. Maypole

On the flipchart write:

- Girl's name
- Boy's name
- Name of a town
- Name of a country
- An animal
- Fruit
- Flower
- Vegetable
- Job/hobby

Taking in sequence each letter of 'Maypole', ask members of the group in turn to give a name beginning with that letter for each category, for example: M = Mabel, Mark, etc. O = Olive, Ollie, etc.

3. Maypole dancing

Give a copy of 'Maypoles' (page 90) to everyone. Ask them to spot the 10 differences between the two pictures.

4. This is a time for fairies, love, enchantment and magic

(Based on *More Mental Aerobics* page 344)

See if the group can turn each of these words into another! List the anagrams, and then the answers, on the flipchart.

SWAP	wasp	NOTE	tone
OCEAN	canoe	PINS	spin
SHIP	hips	EVIL	vile
TABLE	bleat	VOLE	love
GUTS	tugs	SHRUB	brush
DEAR	read	DIRECTOR	creditor
RATE	tear	PIER	ripe
TEAL	late	PALE	leap
SUB	bus	MATE	team
EROS	rose	ROLE	lore

Answers: In right-hand picture – clocks tell different times, tree by church missing, end of cloud added, flag on first tent different, sun's rays missing, flag on second tent different, stripes on pole in reversed spiral, ribbon on girl's plait added, stripes added on dark-haired boy's trousers, flower added

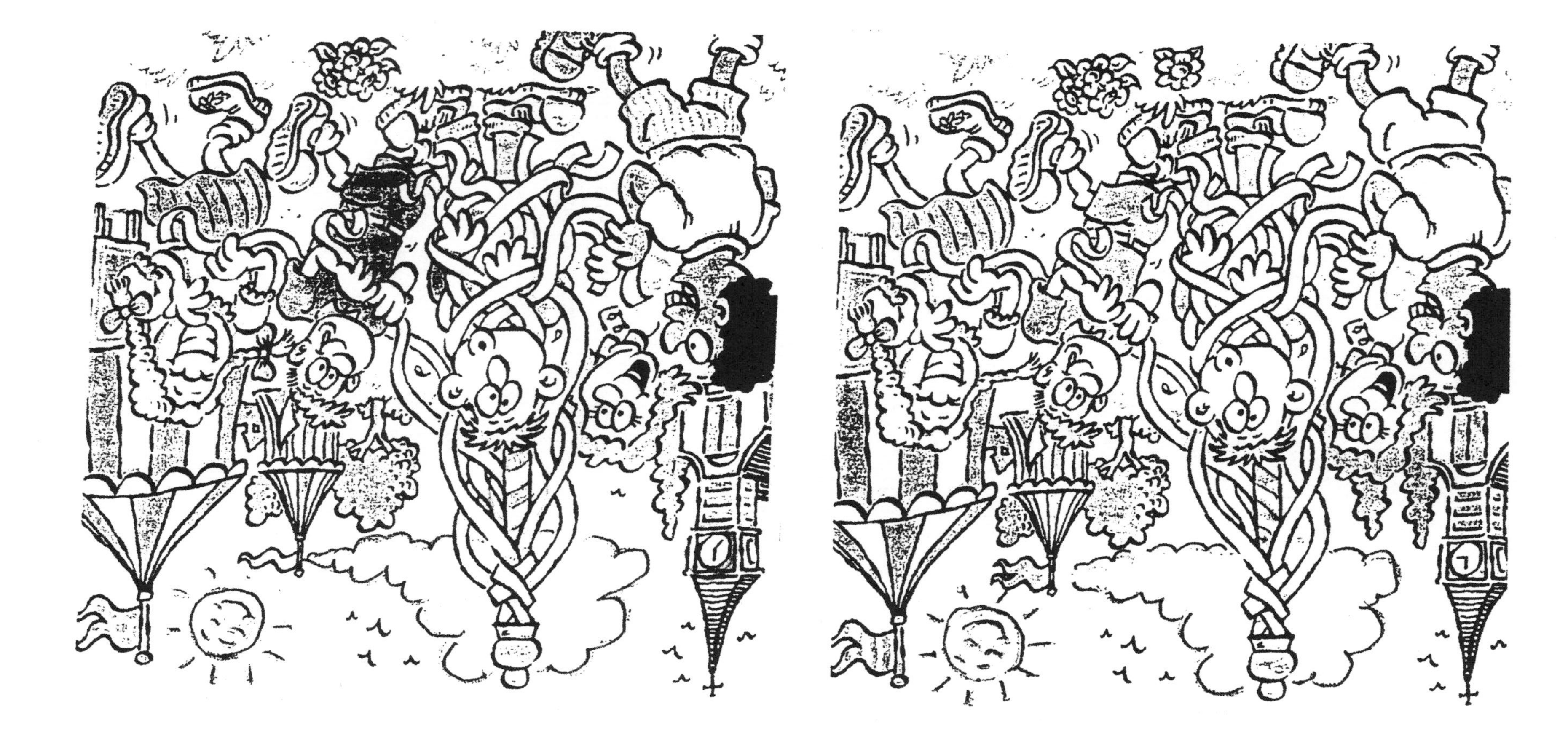

APE	pea	LAPSE	peals
BEARD	bread	SILO	oils
AMEN	name	MADE	mead
RATS	star	FLOW	wolf
TAN	ant	DRAW	ward
BLOW	bowl	TOPS	spot

Add more of your own.

Week 2 – May ball

Equipment: flipchart, pens, paper, dance music, copies of picture quiz on page 94.

1. Reminiscence and discussion

Talk with the group about May balls, has anyone been to one? Or any formal dance? Hunt ball? Graduation ball? Did they get a printed formal invitation? From whom? Can they remember their first dance? Who did they go with? What did they wear? Did they have to sew on lots of sequins? Did they have a special ballgown? Did the men wear white tie and tails, best suits or dinner jackets? Where was it held? How did they travel to the ball? What kind of music did they have? Who played the music? Did anyone go to the tea dances? Who had the last waltz with them? Did they meet their husband/wife at a dance? Was the local dance hall *the* meeting place for young people? Who taught them to dance? Did they have to learn at school for the Christmas Party? Did this entail dancing with the same sex partner around the gym? Anyone have formal dance lessons? Ballet or tap? Did they take part in any shows?

Did anyone watch 'Come Dancing'? Do they remember the formations dancing teams? What does the group think of 'Celebrity Ballroom Dancing'? Do they find it impressive how much effort people have to put in to gain proficiency? Is it obvious who has natural rhythm?

On the flipchart list the different names of local ballrooms and where they were. Are they still there? What is in their place, if not? Also the names of any dance bands the group can think of, local or national. Can they remember any of the singers who went on to become famous?

2. Name that dance

Have the group in turn untangle the dances – write the anagrams on the flipchart. Is anyone willing to demonstrate the steps as each one is solved (including staff!)?

ANGOT	tango	BAAMS	samba
BRMAU	rumba	WOMITELAPTYRSIT	military twostep
LWZTA	waltz	KALOP	polka
PTEUSQIKC	quickstep	CEABRDNNA	barndance
VIJE	jive	LOLRKNDACOR	rock and roll
TOXTOFR	foxtrot	STWIT	twist
AGGRYDNOO	Gay Gordon	BLAEDOASP	pasa doble
HCAACH	cha cha	EP-OBEB	bee-bop
SLATCHERON	Charleston		

3. The hand jive

Sitting in a circle, with suitable music, teach the group how to do this.

4. The Hokey Cokey

Still in a circle, do a sitting-down version of this. When it comes to 'Do the Hokey Cokey and turn around,' say, 'turn your head', and on 'Oh, kiss me in the middle,' say, 'Oh, shake your hands and stamp your feet.'

5. Tea dance

Organise a tea dance. This is a good ice breaker and you will find music is a great way to get people moving without even realising they are being active. Collect old time dance tapes or CDs, make a poster and get everyone to dress up in their best clothes. You could even invite relatives along.

If this is a success it may be something that could be done on a weekly basis.

6. Footsore!

(based on *Language and Word Activities* page 39)

Ask the group in turn. All the answers include 'foot' or 'feet'.

1. Can't dance!...two left feet
2. Lower mountain slopes...foothills
3. A starting position...foothold

4. Settling into a new job...finding your feet
5. Grumpy TV programme...*One Foot in the Grave*
6. Livestock disease that decimated the countryside...foot-and-mouth
7. Embarrassing slip up...putting your foot in it *or* foot in mouth
8. Saying something against yourself...shoot yourself in the foot
9. New Year custom...first-footing
10. Fancy free...footloose
11. Infantryman...foot soldier
12. To have common sense...feet on the ground
13. A salesman may do this...get a foot in the door
14. A nippy dancer has this...fancy footwork
15. Be firm...put your foot down
16. Try your best...best foot forward
17. A mysterious American beast like the Yeti...bigfoot
18. Reel of film...footage
19. Pay the account...foot the bill
20. Theatre illumination...footlights
21. Relax...put your feet up
22. Tentative feline?...pussyfoot

7. The can-can quiz

All the answers begin with the letters 'CAN'.
Ask the group as a whole:

1. A place to eat at work...CANteen
2. A stand for candles...CANdelabra
3. Scottish for 'shrewd'...CANny
4. Small boat with paddles...CANoe
5. One who seeks election...CANdidate
6. Artificial waterway...CANal
7. Container...CANister
8. Frank and open...CANdid
9. Small cage bird...CANary
10. Sugar crystallised by boiling...CANdy
11. To do with dogs...CANine
12. A Swiss state...CANton
13. Floor of a boxing ring...CANvas
14. Sign of the Zodiac...CANcer
15. Capital of Australia...CANberra
16. Kind of cardgame...CANasta
17. A deep gorge...CANyon
18. A person who eats people...CANnibal
19. Plant that is a narcotic...CANnabis
20. A flower...CANdytuft

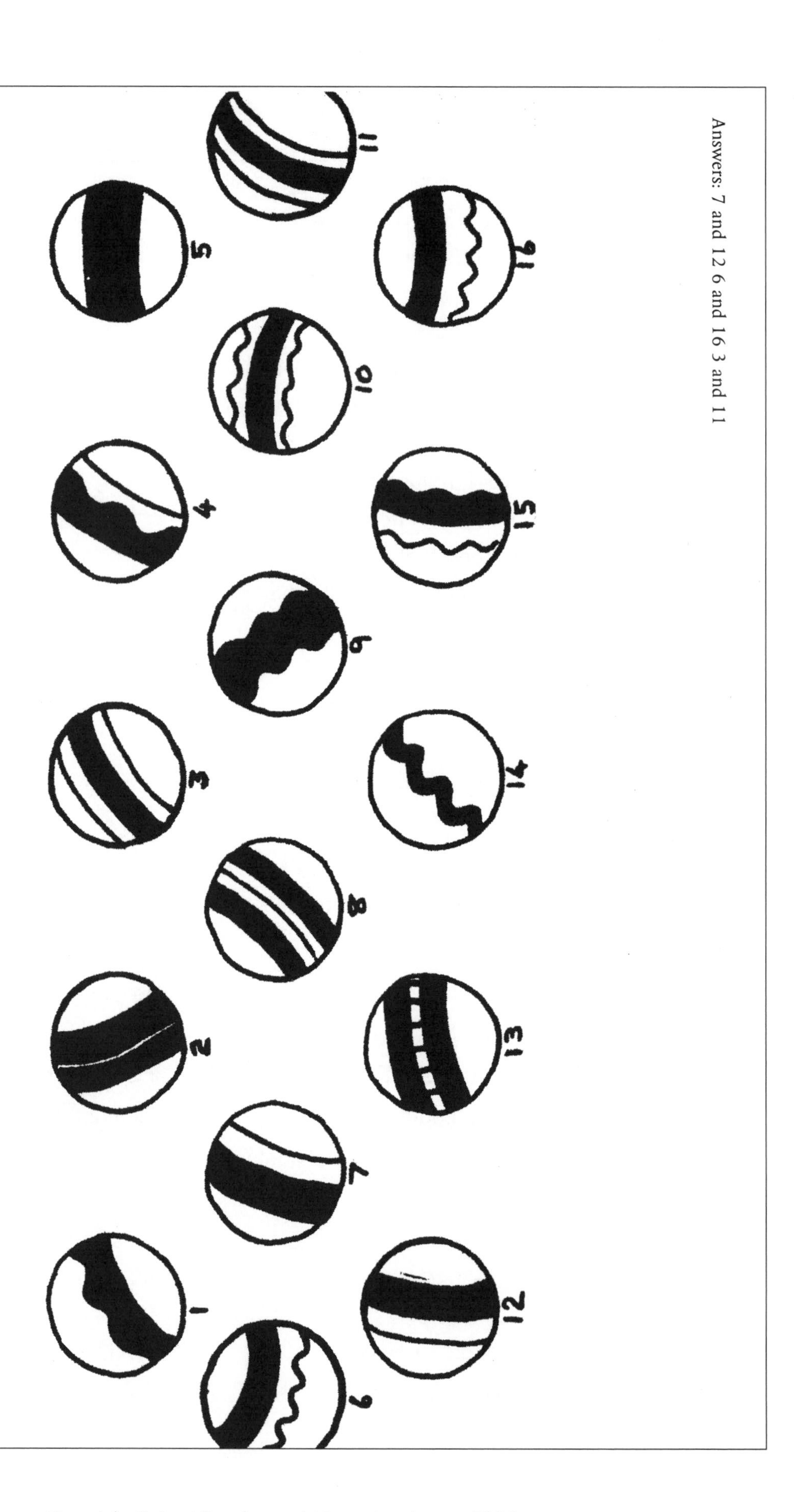
Answers: 7 and 12 6 and 16 3 and 11

8. Fancy-dress balls

Give everyone a copy of the picture on page 94. Match the pairs.

9. See how many words can be found in: WALL FLOWER.

Week 3 – Whitsuntide

Equipment: flipchart, pen, paper.

1. Reminiscence and discussion

Ask the group if Whitsuntide was celebrated in their youth. Did they have Whit walks? The Whitsun parades were led by the local brass band, clergy and local dignitaries, and then the families, with the little girls in their new white dresses. ('Whit' is a corruption of 'White' Sunday). They walked from the church around the town/village to the green or playing field for the 'Whitsun Ale' to begin. Whitsun Ale is a country fair with sports and competitions. The breweries and pubs often sponsored the fair, which is how we came to call beer 'ale'! The Puritans, after the Civil War, banned the Whitsun Ales as a matter of course in their blanket banning of merrymaking, but on the Restoration of King Charles II – who was born on a Whit Monday – they became once more a major social celebration.

Did the ladies in the group have special white dresses when they were young? What did the men wear as boys? Did they attend Sunday school when they were young? Did they go on the Sunday school outings? Where did they go? Do their grandchildren go to Sunday school now? Do they or their family attend church? (Use the following at your discretion to ascertain the wishes of the group re their spiritual preferences: would they like a church representative to visit on a regular basis? On the flipchart list how many different religions – possibly none – are represented in the group. Would they like to have visitors from other faiths?)

In these more secular times the Whitsuntide Bank Holiday has become the Late Spring Bank Holiday. Since it was the first holiday weekend of the year with any hope of fine weather, people would go off to the seaside or countryside – and so we have the first traffic jams of the year! Would the group members go away at this time? What is the longest jam they have encountered? How long did it take to get home? What about delays at airports? Any horror stories about trying to get away for Bank Holiday?

2. It'll be all white

(based on *More Mental Aerobics* page 197)

Ask the group in general. The answers are all connected with white.

1. A fairground ride...white knuckle ride

2. Regal chess pieces...white King and Queen
3. To make clothes white...bleach
4. She had seven little chums...Snow White
5. Blinding snowstorm...whiteout
6. Illegal white powder...cocaine
7. Before coloured TV...black-and-white TV
8. Used for meringues...egg white
9. Where Jack the Ripper prowled...Whitechapel
10. The emblem of Yorkshire...white rose
11. Home of the American President...White House
12. Choppy waves...white caps
13. Born without pigmentation...albino
14. Governmental area of London...Whitehall
15. Dame Vera Lynn sang of these geographical features...white cliffs of Dover
16. The colour brides usually wear...white
17. Slang term for teeth...pearly whites
18. Bing Crosby's seasonal song...'White Christmas'
19. Don't fire until you see...the whites of their eyes
20. What *shade* (pun) you go when scared...as white as a ghost
21. When your team is annihilated by the opposition...a whitewash
22. 'Milky Bars' are made from this...white chocolate
23. If your nickname is 'Chalky' what is your surname?...White
24. A killer fish...great white shark
25. Alice's tardy friend...the White Rabbit

When in traffic jams everyone gets moany and tetchy. Ask the group if they had any games they used to play to help pass the time. If they explain them, play those games.

3. 'I spy with my little eye...'

Make sure everyone has a turn.

4. Traffic 'hangman'

On the flipchart, using only words connected with motor vehicles and motorways.

5. Family car

Give everyone a copy of the spot-the-difference quiz on page 97.

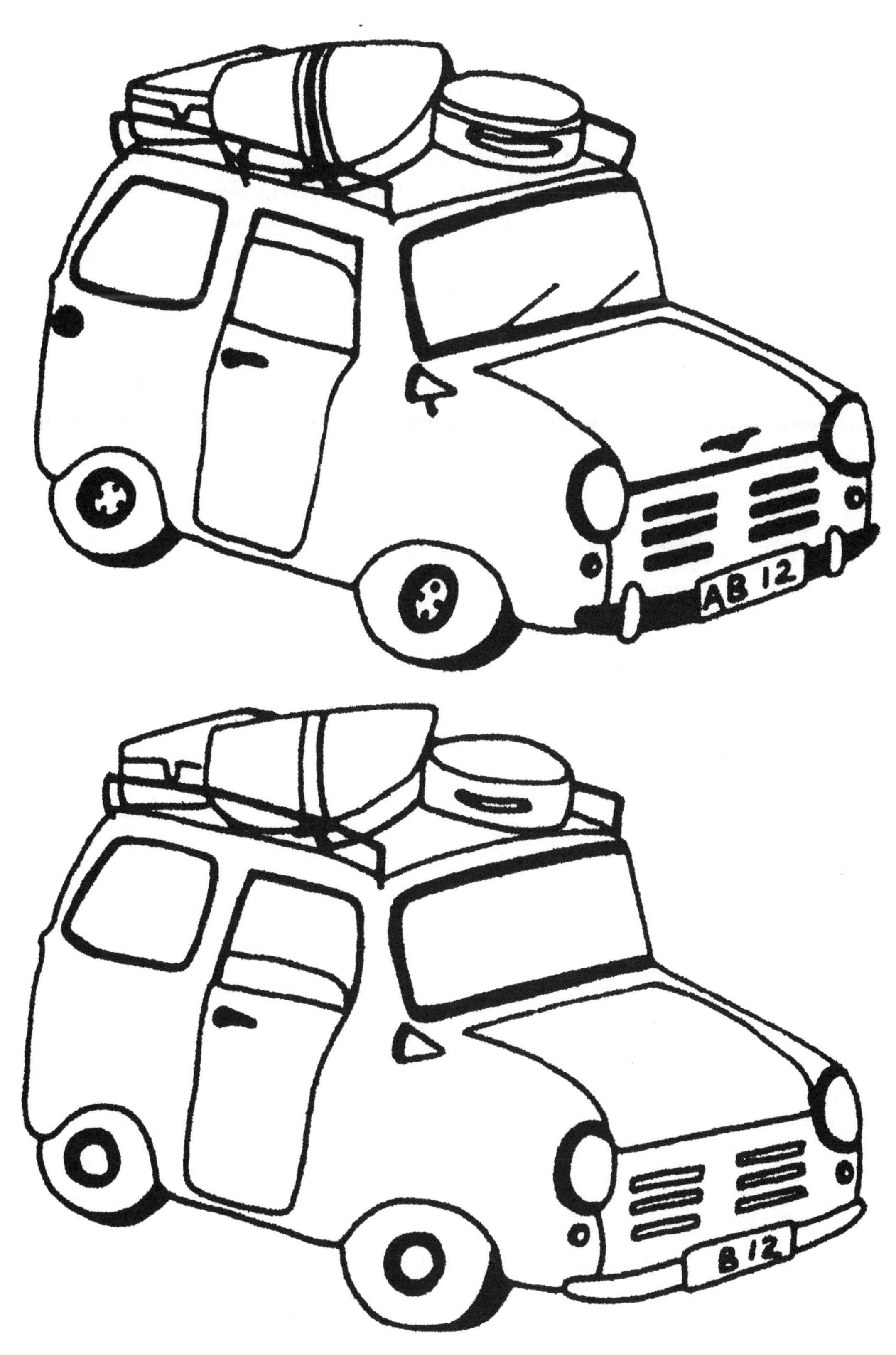

Answers: 1. Hub caps differ 2. Rear door knob missing 3. Case strap different 4. No lid on small case 5. Wind screen wipers missing 6. No badge on bonnet 7. Radiator grills different 8. Side window lower 9. Wing mirror stem missing 10. Different number plates. 11.Bumpers different 12. Strut on roof rack missing 13. Handle on small case different 14. Brackets on bumper missing

6. Sunday school alphabet picnic basket

Begin the game by saying 'In the picnic basket I put **A**pples.' The next person repeats the whole sentence and adds another item '...and a **B**un.'

Go around the group and ask each of them to add another item to the Sunday school picnic basket. They have to remember all the items that went before and add one that begins with the next relevant letter of the alphabet. Remember to get those with the worst memories to begin the game. This encourages support from those with better memories!

7. Motorway food

A nonsense game to encourage invention...

Go round the group and ask each person for the most horrible menu they can think of. It could be made up of the food they hate the most, or an improbable yukky mix.

For example:

Scrambled frogspawn on a leather sole

Snail ice cream

Iced petrol to drink

Or:

Mussels with sprouts

Sago pudding

Gin and tonic

– this is my worst food and drink.

8. See how many words can be made from: BANK HOLIDAY JAMS.

Week 4 – Folklore and customs, legends and myths

Equipment: flipchart, pens, information on any ghosts/haunted houses in the area, *River Dance* video, copies of word search on page 107.

1. Reminiscence and discussion

Folklore is the traditional way people have passed on their history, customs and beliefs. Stories have a power to teach and enthral the young. Talk about maypole dancing – anyone take part? Has anyone seen morris dancing? What was the meaning of the morris dance? – Fertility rites. Perhaps a morris dance troupe could visit? *and* explain why they do it! Pancake racing, Easter egg rolling – did they do these when young? Any local traditions – such as well-dressing in Derbyshire? (Local library/tourist information office will supply information.)

Ask the group which folklore and customs they can remember from their youth? Was there a scary part on the way home that they had to perform a special ritual to get past – like crossing fingers, not standing on the cracks in the pavement, hopping backwards – are there any local superstitions they still observe?

Does anyone have a way of foretelling the weather, such as 'Red sky at night, shepherd's delight, red sky in the morning, sailor's warning', lots of berries signify a harsh winter to come, cows all lying down foretell rain…? Do they remember William Frogatt, the country weather man from Thirsk, who used the signs of nature such as these to forecast weather? He wrote in one of the Sunday papers.

Do group members have a local dialect? Are there any local words they can remember – list them and their meanings. Do some people pronounce the same word differently, depending on where they come from? For example, 'tongue' is *tung* in Yorkshire but *tong* in Lancashire.

Has anyone seen a ghost? Did they have a ghost in their house? Do they know of any haunted houses in the locality? Share info. Did anyone see a fairy when they were young? Do they believe in the little folk? What about leprechauns? Any Irish group members have a story from their youth? Which fairy stories can they still recall?

We have many legends in the UK. Tales of crime and adventure such as Robin Hood, Dick Turpin, King Arthur and the Round Table, also worldwide legendary heroes are known to us, such as Ned Kelly, William Tell, Davy Crockett, Jessie James – add more of your own. We are fascinated by strange creatures such as the Loch Ness Monster, big cats roaming the countryside, mysterious White Horses carved into hillsides, and the famed beauties such as Cleopatra and Helen of Troy – and also by modern 'legends' like Princess Diana, James Dean and Marilyn Monroe.

Ask people to name the national dress of England (beefeater), Ireland (green kilt and sash), Scotland (kilts), Wales (high, pointy hat, long dress). Has anyone worn their national costume? Done their national dance? Perhaps a video of 'River Dance' could be shown to illustrate Irish dancing.

Does anyone have any family traditions? Are they still upheld? Does anyone do any traditional crafts, such as lacemaking, tatting, quiltmaking, weaving, spinning, tapestry, embroidery, knitting, marquetry, woodcarving? If so, could they bring a sample to show the group?

Sometimes nursery rhymes were used to pass on stories and information. For example, 'Ring a ring 'o roses' is supposed to be about the plague, with the ring of red (the roses in the rhyme) being the spots and the 'all fall down' signifying death. 'Pop goes the weasel' refers to the hatters pawning their 'weasels' – a piece of hat-making equipment – to buy food for their families.

2. Nursery rhyme quiz

(from *Mental Aerobics* page 61)

Read a line of a nursery rhyme, and ask the group to say the next line and give the title of the rhyme. Can they still recite the whole rhyme?

When the pie was opened...The birds began to sing.
Sing a song of sixpence

See-saw, Margery Daw...Johnny shall have a new master.
See-saw, Margery Daw

There was a crooked man...Who had a crooked hat.
The crooked sixpence

One shoe off and one shoe on...Diddle, diddle dumpling, my son John.
Diddle, diddle dumpling

With silver buckles on his knee...He'll come back and marry me.
Bobby Shaftoe

Did ever you see such a thing in your life...As three blind mice.
Three Blind Mice

But when she came there...The cupboard was bare.
Old Mother Hubbard

He put her in a pumpkin shell...And there he kept her very well.
Peter, Peter, pumpkin eater

And pulled out a plum...And said, 'What a good boy am I.'
Little Jack Horner

And one for the Dame...And one for the little boy who lives down the lane.
Baa, baa, Black Sheep

To fetch a pail of water...Jack fell down and broke his crown.
Jack and Jill

When she was good...She was very very good.
There was a little girl

She gave them some broth...Without any bread...
There was an old woman who lived in a shoe

Fly away home...Your house is on fire.
Ladybird, ladybird

This little piggy...Went to market...
Five toes

With silver bells and cockle shells...And pretty maids all in a row.
Mary, Mary quite contrary

The clock struck one...The mouse ran down.
Hickory, dickory, dock

He stepped in a puddle...Right up to his middle.
Dr Foster went to Gloucester

To see such sport...And the dish ran away with the spoon.
Hey, diddle diddle

Three men in a tub...And who do you think they be?
Rub-a-dub-dub

And everywhere that Mary went...The lamb was sure to go.
Mary had a little lamb

Sings for his supper...What shall he get? Brown bread and butter.
Little Tommy Tucker

Have lost their mittens...And they began to cry.
Three little kittens

Jack jump over...The candle stick.
Jack, be nimble

Then along came a spider...Who sat down beside her.
Little Miss Muffet

Seven, eight...Lay them straight.
One, two, buckle my shoe

And he called for his bowl...And he called for his fiddlers three.
Old King Cole

What a naughty boy was that...To try to drown poor pussy cat.
Ding, dong bell

The sheep's in the meadow...The cow's in the corn.
Little Boy Blue

Hark, hark...The dogs do bark.
Hark, hark

All the king's horses...And all the king's men.
Humpty Dumpty

I've been up to London to visit the Queen...And what did you there?
Pussycat, Pussycat

Rapping at the window...Crying at the lock...
Wee Willie Winkie

Rings on her fingers...And bells on her toes...
Ride a cock horse to Banbury Cross

Leave them alone and they'll come home...Wagging their tails behind them.
Little Bo-Peep

As I was going to St Ives...I met a man with seven wives.
St Ives

The child who is born on the Sabbath day...Is bonny and blyth and good and gay.
Sunday's child

To buy a fat pig...Home again, home again, jiggety-jig.
To market, to market

She made some tarts...All on a summer's day.
The Queen of Hearts

Met a pie man...Going to the fair...
Simple Simon

Up above the world so high...Like a diamond in the sky...
Twinkle, twinkle, little star

Upstairs and downstairs...And in my lady's chamber...
Goosey, goosey gander

Some like it in the pot...Nine days old.
Pease porridge hot

Sat among the cinders...Warming her pretty little toes...
Little Polly Flinders

His wife could eat no lean...And so betwixt the two of them...
Jack Spratt

3. Muddled proverbs

Folk wisdom was often handed down in proverbs and wise sayings. Can the group complete these proverbs?

1. One good turn...deserves another
2. It never rains but...it pours
3. It takes two to...tango
4. Too many cooks...spoil the broth
5. A stitch in time...saves nine
6. A rolling stone...gathers no moss
7. A barking dog...never bites
8. Honesty...is the best policy
9. The early bird...catches the worm
10. All that glitters...is not gold
11. Curiosity...killed the cat
12. Make hay...while the sun shines
13. Faint heart...never won a fair lady

Complete these proverbs and explain what they are trying to convey.

1. Actions speak...louder than words.
2. All is fair in...love and war.
3. All's well...that ends well.
4. Many a true word...is spoken in jest.
5. An apple a day...keeps the doctor away.
6. Ask no questions...and you'll hear no lies.
7. If you want a thing done well...do it yourself.
8. His bark...is worse than his bite.
9. Beauty is...but skin deep.
10. Better late...than never.
11. Butter wouldn't...melt in his mouth.
12. Children should be seen...and not heard.
13. It's no use crying...over spilt milk.
14. Cut your coat...according to your cloth.
15. Discretion is the...better part of valour.
16. It is an ill wind...that blows nobody any good.
17. Jack of all trades...and master of none.
18. Every cloud...has a silver lining.
19. Kill two birds...with one stone.
20. You can't teach...an old dog new tricks.

4. Find the proverb

The letter in each of the four intertwined shapes make a word. The four words make a well known saying. (*Answer*: Least said soonest mended)

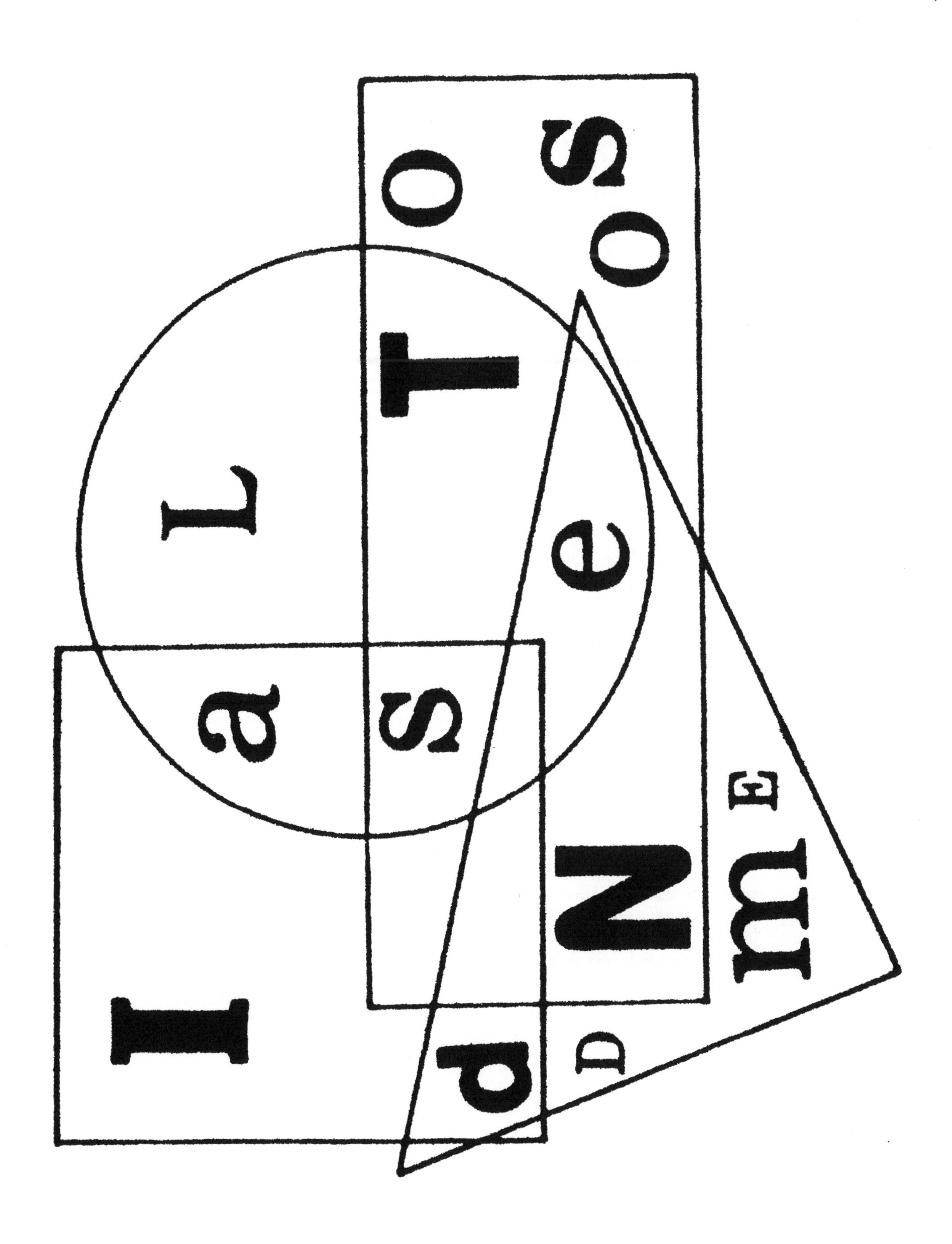

5. Wise words

(from *More Mental Aerobics* page 138.)

Complete these well known nuggets of wisdom! Read out one half of each maxim and let the group supply the rest.

1. He who hesitates...is lost.
2. Nothing ventured...nothing gained.
3. Hope springs eternal...in the human breast.
4. When ignorance is bliss...'tis folly to be wise.
5. What you don't know...can't hurt you.
6. It is no use flogging...a dead horse.
7. Let sleeping dogs...lie.
8. The child is the father...of the man.
9. Fools rush in...where angels fear to tread.
10. An eye for an eye...and a tooth for a tooth.
11. To err is human...to forgive, divine.
12. A little learning...is a dangerous thing.
13. The Lord helps...those who help themselves.
14. Look before...you leap.
15. Turn...the other cheek.
16. If at first you don't succeed...try, try, try again.
17. Forgive...and forget.
18. Absence...makes the heart grow fonder.
19. To do...or die.
20. Out of sight...out of mind.
21. More haste...less speed.
22. If winter comes...can spring be far behind?
23. Beauty is truth...and truth is beauty.
24. Tis better to have loved and lost...than never to have loved at all.
25. 'O wad some pow'r the giftie gie us'...'Tae see ourselves as ithers see us.'
26. As Del-Boy says, 'He who dares'...WINS.

6. Myths, tales and legends quiz

(based on *More Mental Aerobics* page 57)

This is a long quiz which could be spread over a few days. In teams named after a legendary figure (perhaps 'Robin Hood and his Merry Men', 'King Arthur and the Knights of the Round Table') answer the following questions:

1. Who slayed the dragon and is England's patron saint?...St George
2. Where did Robin and his Merry Men live?...Sherwood Forest
3. Which king pulled Excalibur from the stone?...Arthur
4. Who climbed the beanstalk?...Jack
5. On which night do witches fly?...Halloween
6. Which King burned the cakes?...Alfred
7. Who killed Cock Robin?...Sparrow
8. Who was Hansel's sister?...Gretel
9. Who turned everything he touched to gold?...King Midas
10. Who lived in Transylvania?...Count Dracula
11. Who was Sundance's partner?...Butch Cassidy
12. Who went with Jason to find the fleece?...The Argonauts
13. Who fell when he flew too near the sun?...Icarus
14. Who was at the centre of the labyrinth?...The Minotaur
15. How did Cleopatra die?...she was bitten by an asp.
16. Who had a magic hammer that returned to his hand when thrown?...Thor
17. Who was King Arthur's wife?...Guinevere
18. Who wrote 'The Ugly Duckling' and other fairy stories?...Hans Christian Andersen
19. In which play are there three witches?...*Macbeth*
20. Who had snakes for hair?...Medusa
21. Who shot an apple from his son's head?...William Tell
22. Who couldn't turn the tide?...King Canute
23. Who is the Roman god of love?...Cupid
24. Who had to hold up the sky?...Atlas
25. Who has a famous 'belt' in the stars?...Orion
26. Where is the home of the Abominable Snowman?...the Himalayas
27. Who finished his game of bowls?...Sir Francis Drake

28. What was released from Pandora's box?...evil spirits and woe
29. Who came out of her box last and saved the world?...Hope
30. How did Theseus find his way out of the labyrinth?...Ariadne gave him a ball of thread which he unravelled to mark his way
31. What is the name of the three-headed dog at the gates of Hades?...Cerberus
32. Who was the famous Greek hero of the Trojan War?...Achilles
33. How was he killed?...shot in the heel with an arrow
34. What was William Bonney better known as?...Billy the Kid
35. Who fell in love with his own reflection?...Narcissus
36. Who loved him in vain?...Echo
37. It is said an Irish giant threw a sod of earth at a Scottish giant, it landed in the sea and became an island – which one?...Arran
38. Who pursued Moby Dick?...Captain Ahab
39. The heroine of Lewis Carroll's books was?...Alice
40. Where was King Arthur's court?...Camelot
41. Who was the companion of Robinson Crusoe?...Man Friday
42. Who did Professor Higgins turn into a lady?...Eliza Doolittle
43. *My Fair Lady* was the musical version of which novel by Bernard Shaw?...*Pygmalion*
44. Who murdered his many wives?...Bluebeard
45. Who told the tales of Brer Rabbit?...Uncle Remus
46. What was Ali Baba's magic password?...'Open Sesame'
47. Who didn't 'give a damn'?...Rhett Butler
48. Who was Winnie the Pooh's chum?...Christopher Robin
49. Which Frenchman was known for his extremely long nose?...Cyrano de Bergerac
50. Who was the tragic wife of Othello?...Desdemona
51. This Spanish hero had a way with the ladies...Don Juan
52. Who married Mr Rochester?...Jane Eyre
53. Who trained Oliver to be a pickpocket?...Fagin
54. Which poor monster was constructed from body parts?...Frankenstein
55. Who is Mark Twain's most famous hero?...Huckleberry Finn
56. Who rode naked through Coventry?...Lady Godiva
57. Who spied on her?...Peeping Tom
58. This little Swiss girl lived in the Alps with her grandfather?...Heidi

59. Whose face launched a thousand ships?...Helen of Troy
60. Who was the hero of Sir Walter Scott's novel which was televised?...Ivanhoe
61. What were the names of the man who could change his personality?...Dr Jekyll/Mr Hyde
62. Who is the Queen of the Fairies?...Titania
63. Name the gorgon who could change you to stone with a look...Medusa
64. The hero of *The Jungle Book* was...Mowgli
65. The mountain on which the Greek gods lived...Olympia
66. The Roman god of the sea...Neptune
67. The boy who didn't want to grow up...Peter Pan
68. The winged horse was...Pegasus
69. How did Dorothy get home from Oz?...she clicked the heels of her Red Shoes together
70. Whose nose grows when he fibs?...Pinocchio
71. Which legendary twins founded Rome?...Romulus and Remus
72. Who was raised by apes in the jungle?...Tarzan
73. Who had seven little chums?...Snow White
74. Can you name them?...Sneezy, Dopey, Happy, Doc, Grumpy, Sleepy, Bashful
75. Where do the Lost Boys live?...Nevernever Land
76. Who is the miserly man in *A Christmas Carol*?...Scrooge
77. Who is Bambi's friend?...Thumper
78. Who was not at all brave in Oz?...the Cowardly Lion
79. Who rid Hamelin of rats?...The Pied Piper
80. Tarzan's sidekick was named after a big cat, but was a primate!...Cheetah
81. A talking scarecrow...Worzel Gummidge
82. The fairy in *Peter Pan*...Tinkerbell

7. Nursery rhymes and legends word search

A	L	A	D	D	I	N	B	A	T	E	R
L	K	O	T	D	T	Z	V	J	B	T	V
I	N	A	R	Q	D	I	E	N	A	A	I
C	C	A	E	U	D	E	X	O	L	R	W
E	E	G	O	O	A	T	U	R	U	Z	B
B	R	D	G	E	O	S	U	R	C	A	N
L	S	C	R	O	O	G	E	F	A	N	I
U	A	S	U	D	E	M	N	I	R	M	G
E	J	A	K	C	A	L	B	K	D	O	A
R	O	B	I	N	S	O	N	P	K	P	F
F	R	A	N	K	E	N	S	T	E	I	N
G	U	I	N	E	V	E	R	E	G	D	O

Can you find these characters?

DRACULA, ALADDIN, ALICE, FRANKENSTEIN, BLUEBEARD, GODIVA, GUINEVERE, ROBINSON CRUSOE, SCROOGE, FAGIN, TARZAN, MEDUSA...plus the hidden witch's familiar (BLACK CAT)

8. See how many words can you make from: MYTHS AND LEGENDS.

Activities for June

Week 1 – The weather

Equipment: flipchart, pens, paper.

1. Reminiscence and discussion

This topic is world famous as the only conversation with which the British are comfortable... Does the group think this is because our weather is so changeable? Ask the group if they think the weather has changed since they were young...how? Do they feel this is really so, or does the memory tend to remember only the best and worst times we experienced...e.g. that single, long, hot summer when we played out every day, or that one awful winter when we were snowed in? Ask the group in turn to name their favourite and worst type of weather, and their reasons for the choice.

Can anyone foretell the weather? Do they feel the damp in their bones? Can they smell snow coming or feel the change in air pressure that heralds a thunderstorm? Do they feel that the weather influences their mood? Anyone suffer from SAD (Seasonal Affective Disorder)? Think about the poor folk in Norway, etc., who have almost permanent night time in the winters. Do they all feel happier when the sun shines, and a bit down in miserable weather? Has anyone ever been flooded? What happened? How did they cope? Were they insured? Does the group remember the awful flash flood that devastated Boscastle? Does anyone know the official term for hitting a waterlogged road at speed (aquaplaning)?

Conversely, can they remember the droughts when there was a hosepipe ban and standpipes, and when some people in Yorkshire had water delivered in tankers, and how the reservoirs were low enough to expose the villages that had been sacrificed to build them? This was especially evident at Ladybower Reservoir in Derbyshire (where the Dambuster pilots practised the bouncing bomb techniques in World War II). How did the group conserve water? Only boil enough water for one cup of tea/coffee at a time? Did they share a bath? Not flush the toilet every time? Put a brick in the cistern to reduce amount of water needed to fill it? Have rainwater tubs connected to their drainpipes? How did their gardens fare? Did they catch people cheating and watering gardens or washing cars? What do they think about the scandal of all the Water Boards' leaking pipes? Are they still careful about conserving water?

Is the group afraid of thunderstorms? What scares them most – the thunder or the lightning? How do they cope with this fear? Did they inherit it from their parents? What is the safest way to protect yourself in a thunderstorm? Don't stand under a tree. Has any member of the group ever been lost in a fog? What is a particularly dense fog called? (A peasouper.) Can anyone remember smog? What caused this to form? (Smoke and fog.) Why do we not suffer from this nowadays? – Because the Clean Air Act prevented factories from belching out noxious smoke and created smoke-free zones where only smokeless fuel could be burnt. Smog caused many respiratory diseases – can people remember how they tried to avoid this? (Smog masks and scarves over mouths – they were soon covered in black, sooty deposits.)

Snow and ice are the most dangerous types of weather for older people as they cause fractures to wrists and femurs. Any hints on how to avoid slips? (Good boots with grips, avoid going out in ice and snow – shops will often deliver or ask neighbours for assistance. Do not rush anywhere.) Does the group have any tips on keeping warm? Did the ladies all wear vests *and* liberty bodices when they young? Remember those rubber buttons! Good advice is to start the day with a good bowl of porridge, wear layers, always wear a hat, as most heat is lost from head, and keep feet and hands warm.

As summer is fast approaching it is a good time to discuss protecting skin from the sun because of the increased risk of skin cancer – it is especially important as we get older, as our skin becomes more fragile and thinner. A hat is a good protector, sit in the shade, avoid the midday sun and drink lots of water. It is easy to become dehydrated and not realise, as often we are already dehydrated when we first feel thirsty. Has anyone been sunburnt? Had heat-stroke? Does the group think we are feeling the effects of global warming?

Can the group remember the colours of the rainbow? Do they know a mnemonic (pronounced 'nemonic') for remembering the order? **R**ichard **O**f **Y**ork **G**ave **B**attle **I**n **V**ain = **R**ed **O**range, **Y**ellow, **G**reen, **B**lue, **I**ndigo, **V**iolet.

2. Weather forecasting folklore

On the flipchart write down all the ways the group can think of to forecast weather – for example, observing changes in pinecones or a piece of seaweed. Recall sayings such as:

- Red sky at night, shepherd's delight.
- Red sky in the morning, shepherd's warning.
- Mackerel sky, mackerel sky – never long wet, never long dry.
- The higher the clouds, the better the weather.
- Rain before seven, clear by eleven.
- When dew is on the grass no rain will come to pass.
- When seagulls come inland it is stormy at sea.
- Rainbow in the morning, travellers take warning.

- Rainbow at night, traveller's delight.
- When a halo rings the moon or sun, rain's approaching at a run.
- Moss dry, sunny sky, moss wet, rain we'll get.
- Cows lying down means it will rain.
- Bees do not swarm before a storm.

Often people – especially William Foggatt from Thirsk (does the group remember his predictions in *The People*?) – see the behaviour of animals, such as squirrels collecting and hiding lots of nuts, or natural signs, like lots of berries on the trees, as a sign of a hard winter to come and early appearances of swifts and swallows as heralding a good summer. Any others? Does anyone in the group have a barometer? Here are some rhymes for them:

When the glass falls low,
Stand by for a blow.
When it slowly rises high,
All the light sails you may fly.
Fast rise after low
Foretells a stronger blow.

3. Weather songs

On the flipchart list all the songs/music the group can think of concerning weather. Ask them to sing or hum a little of each. Some suggestions:

- Singing in the Rain
- You are my Sunshine
- Bring me Sunshine
- The Sunshine of your Smile
- The Sun has got his Hat on
- April Showers
- Blow the Wind Southerly
- Thunder and Lightning Polka
- Somewhere over the Rainbow
- Let it Snow
- The Little White Cloud that Cried
- Stormy Weather
- Frosty the Snowman
- The Snowman (Aled Jones' version).

4. Stormy weather – anagrams of weather conditions

Write the anagrams on the flipchart and give everyone paper to write the solutions.

SHUERNRACI	hurricanes	OOTRNAD	tornado
WSNO	snow	ALIH	hail
SCDLUO	clouds	ROSDIARTS	stair rods
GOF	fog	RSAOBI	isobar
RSTOF	frost	NUS	sun
DADTASSNOGC	cats and dogs	LAGE	gale
NIAR	rain	GNNIGLTIH	lightning
RTHUDEN	thunder	WEELRZBEFGINO	below freezing
SSUNEIHN	sunshine	LICECI	icicle
DOOLF	flood		

5. What am I?

(based on *Mental Aerobics* page 265)

In teams named after weather conditions. A nominated person from each team gives the answer after discussion. All the answers are to do with weather.

Score three points if guessed straightaway, two after two clues, one after all clues given.

1. City gents carry me.
   I can fit in a handbag.
   I have spokes.
   umbrella (Why do city gents carry umbrellas? Because they can't walk!)

2. am frozen.
   I used to be rain.
   If I hit you I am painful.
   hail

3. I turn the mill sails.
   When I come from the North I can bring snow.
   March is my favourite month.
   wind

9. Ladies of the past made great 'play' with me.
   I am mostly used in hot weather.
   I create a little breeze.
   fan

10. I sit on high.
    My points make NEWS.
    I usually have a cockerel on me.
    weather vane

11. I am very complicated to set up.
    I prefer stripes.
    I am found on beaches and in gardens.
    deckchair

4. I need to be 'blocked'.
People enjoy my getting up and going down.
Without me nothing can live.
sun

5. I am made of sun and rain.
I am colourful.
I may have gold at my end.
rainbow

6. I was named for a general.
I make puddle jumping fun.
In the counties I have a green brigade.
Wellington

7. I am in the garden.
I am a saver of a precious resource.
I am attached to a drainpipe.
water butt

8. I am sensitive to pressure.
I usually hang around in halls.
People give me a good tap.
barometer

12. I am moist.
I block vision.
A horn accompanies me.
fog

13. I can be white or black.
Evaporation makes me.
I have Latin names for my shapes.
clouds

14. Sometimes glamour girls rather then scientists present me.
My accuracy is often questioned.
I follow the News.
weather forecast

15. I can be forked.
I can strike.
I am electrically charged.
lightning

16. In German I am the name of one of Santa's reindeer.
I am half the name of a famous polka.
My clouds are very black.
thunder

Add more of your own.

6. See how many words can be made from: WEATHER FORECAST.

Week 2 – Dog days

Perhaps a representative from Mountain Rescue, Guide Dogs for the Blind, Hearing Dogs or a police dog handler could visit to demonstrate their dog's skills, or maybe a member of staff could bring in a dog who likes to be patted.

Equipment: flipchart, paper, pens, copies of word search (page 116) and picture quiz (page 117).

1. Reminiscence and discussion

Ask the group if any of them had a dog when they were young. What breed was it? What was its name? Did they have sole responsibility for its care? Did they train it? Any funny stories or adventures with their dog? Does anyone still own a dog? Did anyone have a cat when they were young? Called? How long did it live? Do they still have one? What peculiar characteristics did their cat have? Did anyone have a different kind of pet? (List.) Does anyone *not* like pets?

Ask the group if they can recall the names of the two charities that support pets (RSPCA and PDSA). Do they know what these acronyms stand for? (Royal Society for the Prevention of Cruelty to Animals and People's Dispensary for Sick Animals.) Discuss man's cruelty to animals. Does the group think the British are more kind to pets than other nations? How does this square with the overflowing rescue centres like Battersea Dogs' Home? How would the group feel about eating dogs, as the Chinese do? (These are dogs specially bred for eating, kept much like chickens, and are a great delicacy that only the very rich can afford. The ordinary Chinese in China love their dogs very much, they are expensive to buy and expensive to keep.)

Has anyone been a member of, or raised funds for, animal charities? Which ones? Does anyone support Guide Dogs for the Blind? What did they used to save for them? (Silver paper.) Has anyone ever seen a guide dog working? Can the group think of other jobs a dog can do? (Hearing dogs, sniffer dogs (drugs, bodies and explosives), dogs who can detect signs of an epileptic fit before the sufferer and enable them to lie somewhere safely, or who are able to detect cancers, search and rescue dogs, police dogs, guard dogs, sheep and cattle dogs, huskies.)

Does the group enjoy watching Crufts? Are there some breeds of dogs that the group really dislike? Why? Are they impressed with the obedience training? Can the group remember Barbara Woodhouse? Do they think owners grow to resemble their dogs? What does the group think about pampered pets? Discuss the fashionable clothes and jewels they are put into by their owners. (Some pictures would be interesting.) What about those people who leave a fortune to a cat or dog? Does the group think that dogs are 'man's best friend' or do they prefer the very selective affection sometimes given us by cats?

2. Doggie breeds

(based on *More Mental Aerobics* page 176)

On the flipchart list as many breeds as the group can think of. Suggestions:

Jack Russell	Foxhound	Pomeranian
Yorkshire Terrier	Pekinese	Cocker Spaniel
Wire-haired Fox Terrier	Basset Hound	Old English Sheepdog
Cairn Terrier	Dalmatian	Doberman Pinscher
Airedale Terrier	Alsatian	Afghan Hound

Bedlington Terrier	Bulldog	Dachshund
Chihuahua	Mastiff	Great Dane
Rottweiler	Greyhound	Red setter
St Bernard	Beagle	Poodle: standard, miniature, toy
Labrador	Whippet	King Charles Spaniel
Golden Retriever	Chow	Newfoundland
Welsh Corgi	Boxer	Irish Wolfhound
Border Collie	Husky	Bloodhound
Scottish Terrier	Shihtzu	Pharaoh Hound

3. Doggie quiz

Ask the group in general.

1. A film starring many dogs!...*101 Dalmatians*
2. Which collie always came home?...Lassie
3. A Royal favourite...Corgi
4. Another name for the Alsatian...German Shepherd
5. Surprisingly this breed used to help the French bring in the fishing nets!...Poodle
6. Which breed brings brandy when you are lost?...St Bernard
7. Do dogs have colour vision?...no
8. The young of a dog is a...puppy
9. The female is called a...bitch
10. Were dogs in service during the war?...yes, as Red Cross dogs and mine detectors
11. What is a cross-bred dog called?...mongrel or Heinz 57!
12. A pure bred is a...pedigree
13. Who was Mickey Mouse's dog?...Pluto
14. A cartoon dog with protruding teeth...Goofy
15. What breed is Snoopy?...Beagle
16. What breed is Fred?...Basset Hound
17. What was the title of the sad song about a boy and his dog?...'Old Shep'
18. The dog in the 'Wooden Tops' was called...Spotty Dog
19. A nodding dog who sells insurance...Churchill
20. The dog in Enid Blyton's *Famous Five*...Timmy

Add more of your own.

4. Doggy expressions

List on the flipchart as many as the group can think of. Some prompts:

- sick as a dog
- let sleeping dogs lie
- raining cats and dogs
- man's best friend
- dog tired
- dog days
- double dog dare
- top dog
- going to the dogs
- as the dog returns to its vomit (Biblical)
- as faithful as a puppy
- lap dog
- lying hound/cur
- doggone it
- sun dog (a parhelion or mock sun formed by reflection of sunlight in ice crystals in cirrus clouds)

5. Millionaire dog

In teams, ask the Millionaire-type questions, listing all possible answers. Begin with Team 1, at the first wrong answer ask Team 2 and carry on the questions with them. (Correct answers are in bold type.)

1. What is the colour of a Westie?...black, chocolate, black and tan, **white**
2. What are the three colours of Labradors?...black, white and rowan/blue, black, white and tan; black, white and red; **yellow, black and chocolate**
3. Which food is the healthiest for dogs' teeth?...fresh beef/chicken, biscuits, tinned meat, **dry food**
4. Which film starred a St Bernard?...*Scooby Doo*, *Cats and Dogs*, *Paws*, **Beethoven**
5. What breed was Mr Woo in Coronation Street?...Greyhound, Border Collie, Yorkie, **Shihtzu**
6. What breed is a Jack Russell?...**terrier**, gundog, toy, working breed
7. What is another name for an Alsatian?...Rottweiler, Collie, Doberman, **German shepherd**
8. What is the Queen's favourite breed?...**Corgi**, Bulldog, Pit Bull, Staffordshire
9. Name the two types of Corgi...**Cardigan and Pembroke**, Welsh and Cardigan, Pembroke and Argyll, Welsh and Pembroke
10. What colour is the Weirmasener?...yellow, black, black and tan, **silver grey**
11. Which king was a breed named after?...Elvis, Henry VIII, Charles I, **Charles II**
12. Which breed advertises 'Hush Puppies'?...Springer Spaniel, Cocker Spaniel, Husky, **Basset Hound**
13. Which vaccination is required for a dog to stay in kennels?...parvo virus, whooping cough, **kennel cough**, dry cough
14. What is the maximum number of litters a bitch can have before she must have a year's rest?...3, 4, **5**, 6

6. Lost dogs

S	P	A	N	I	E	L	H	T	J
H	I	B	O	X	E	R	O	E	A
E	B	E	A	G	L	E	U	R	M
L	D	O	F	O	O	F	N	R	T
T	H	H	D	X	F	O	D	I	G
I	N	D	B	I	W	W	H	E	I
E	M	L	T	E	R	L	W	R	G
L	S	S	H	U	S	K	Y	L	R
A	A	E	S	A	C	N	D	N	O
M	B	U	L	L	D	O	G	M	C

Can you find the following lost dogs?

MASTIFF, CORGI, SHELTIE, SPANIEL, BOXER, BULLDOG, HOUND, BEAGLE, HUSKY, TERRIER

7. Give a dog a name

Give everyone a copy of the quiz on page 117 and ask them to match the pictures to the breed names.

8. See how many words can be made from: BATTERSEA DOGS HOME.

Labrador	Sheepdog	St Bernard	Basset Hound	Yorkshire Terrier	Alsatian	Bulldog
Cairn	Poodle	Bloodhound	Bull Terrier	Boxer	Fox Terrier	Chihuahua
Dachshund	Spaniel	Dalmatian	Corgi	Chow	Pekinese	King Charles

Answers: 1. Pekinese 2. Alsatian 3 Cairn 4. Bloodhound 5. Dachshund 6. Bull terrier 7. Corgi 8. Spaniel 9. Chow 10. Labrador 11. Bassett hound 12. Chihuahua 13. Boxer 14. Yorkshire Terrier 15. King Charles 16. Sheepdog 17. St Bernard 18. Fox terrier 19. Poodle 20. Bulldog 21. Dalmatian

Week 3 – The stars and the moon in June

Equipment: flipchart, paper, pens, collection of astrological predictions from various newspapers/magazines, pictures of signs of the zodiac (cut out from magazine, enlarge, and laminate if possible), science fiction space video (*Star Wars*, *Star Trek*, etc.).

1. Reminiscence and discussion

Talk with the group about the moon and stars. Does anyone know any of the constellations? Can they find them in the night sky? Can the group give all three names of the most recognisable grouping? (The Plough, *Ursa Major* or the Big Dipper – the last American, as the shape looks like the implement the settlers used to get water from the bucket.) There is also the similar, smaller constellation close by, the Little Plough, *Ursa Minor* or Little Dipper. (NB *ursa* is Latin for 'bear'). Did any of the group go out stargazing when they were young? When is the best time to see the stars? (Clear, frosty nights.)

Can the group remember watching the first moon landing on TV? What do they think about the conspiracy theorists who don't believe it happened and that it was filmed in a quarry, like *Dr Who*? Can the group remember the sputniks? What was the name of the dog the Russians sent into orbit? (Little Lemon.) And then the first man in space? (Yuri Gagarin.) What do they think about all the satellites now orbiting the Earth? Have they ever seen them passing overhead?

Does the group enjoy science fiction? Would they like to watch a video? Which?

On the flipchart, list all the science fiction books/films they have enjoyed or can remember – *Dr Who, Star Wars, ET, Star Trek, War of the Worlds, Journey into Space* (radio series), Jules Verne's *Time Machine*, etc.

Can the group name the planets in our solar system? Write them on flipchart then ask for them to be put in the correct order of distance from the Sun (sun–mercury–venus–earth–mars–jupiter–saturn–uranus–neptune–pluto). There *may* be a further planet after Pluto. Can they say which have rings around them? (Saturn, Uranus, Neptune.) Who was the planet Mars named after? (Mars, the God of War, because it is the Red Planet and reminiscent of blood. Its two moons are called after his dogs, Phobos (meaning 'fear') and Deimos (meaning 'panic').)

The nearest celestial body to us is the moon, which has had a great influence on mankind. Because of its gravitational pull, it controls the tides. The moon takes 28 days to circle the Earth and its shape appears to change with changes in the amount of its illuminated surface facing us. The various shapes are known as...

THE PHASES OF THE MOON

- *crescent moon* – is 'sickle-shaped', before or after a half-moon
- *gibbous moon* – is between a full moon and a half-moon in shape

- *half-moon* – looks like half a circle. Sometimes called a quarter moon, meaning that the moon has completed one quarter of an orbit around the Earth from either the full or new moon position
- *new moon* – is the phase of the moon when it is not visible from the Earth, as the side facing towards us is not lit by the sun
- *a waxing moon* – grows larger from *right* to *left* as it becomes a crescent, a half, a gibbous, and finally a full moon
- *a waning moon* – grows less from *left* to *right*
- *the full moon* – appears as a full circular disc in the sky. It is given different names at different times of year. Ask the group if they can think of reasons for the different names:

January	Moon After Yule, Wolf Moon, Old Moon
February	Snow Moon, Hunger Moon
March	Sap Moon, Crow Moon, Lenten Moon
April	Grass Moon, Egg Moon
May	Milk Moon, Planting Moon
June	Rose Moon, Flower Moon, Strawberry Moon
July	Thunder Moon, Hay Moon
August	Grain Moon, Green Corn Moon
September	Fruit Moon, Harvest Moon
October	Harvest Moon, Hunter's Moon
November	Hunter's Moon, Frosty Moon, Beaver Moon
December	Moon Before Yule, Long Night Moon

Blue moon – When two full Moons appear in a single month, the second one is called a 'blue moon' – this happens every two and half years.

The **Man in the Moon**, carrying a bundle of twigs or a bucket, has been seen for centuries. Folklore says he was a beggar who collected firewood on a Sunday and so was banished to the moon as a punishment, to live a perpetual **Mon**day on the Moon. Does the group have any other explanations? Were they told the Moon was made of green cheese when they were little?

2. Moonstruck

In teams named after planets, ask the group to write the answers to this lunar quiz. Exchange papers to mark answers. Give both answers; the correct one is in bold type.

1. Is the Moon bigger or smaller than the Earth?...bigger or **smaller**
2. What are the circular features on the Moon's surface?...oceans or **craters**
3. Does the same side of the moon always face the Earth?...**yes** or no

4. How far away is the moon from Earth?...238,900 miles or **1,238,900 miles**
5. Does the Moon have an atmosphere?...yes or **no**
6. Who was the first person to walk on the Moon?...**Neil Armstrong** or John Glenn
7. When was the first Moon walk?...**1969** or 1965
8. How long does it take the Moon to revolve around the Earth?...**1 month** or 1 year
9. On the Moon would you feel lighter or heavier than on Earth?...**lighter** or heavier
10. On the Moon would the sky look blue or black?...blue or **black**

3. Moonlight sonata

How many songs to do with the Moon can the group think of, and maybe sing?

List on flipchart. Suggestions:

- Paper Moon
- Everyone's Gone to the Moon
- Under the Moon of Love
- By the Light of the Silvery Moon
- Carolina Moon
- Shine on Harvest Moon
- Fly me to the Moon
- Moon River
- Moonraker (from the James Bond film)
- East of the Sun, West of the Moon
- Hey Diddle Diddle, the Cat and the Fiddle,...the cow jumped over the MOON!

4. It's in the stars

Ask everyone their star sign and read their alleged prediction from today's paper. Do they regularly look at their stars? Do they believe them? Compare the predictions in different newspapers/magazines. Does the group only believe the good fortune?

Ask if members of the group agree with the supposed traits of their star sign, and did the jobs they had match?

Aquarius, the Water Carrier (21 January – 19 February) – brilliant, visionary, curious, open-minded, original, independent and eccentric. Emotionally detached but sociable, more intellectual than practical. *Professions*: inventing, research, social organising or activism, astrology, communications, computer sciences, electronics. *Famous Aquarians*: Charles Dickens, Ronald Reagan, Mia Farrow, Galileo, James Dean.

Pisces, the Two Fishes (20 February – 20 March) – sensitive, emotional, sunny, impressionable, dreamy, creative, psychic, mystical, can be evasive and deceitful, good listener, adaptable, sympathetic, sees both sides, can be delicate and vulnerable under stress, but capable of great strength. *Professions*: music, dance, film, charitable work, counselling, jobs involving water, chemicals, oil, drugs, nursing, clergy. *Famous Pisceans*: Chopin, Liz Taylor, Einstein, Edward Kennedy, Michelangelo, Rex Harrison.

Aries, the Ram (21 March – 19 April) – assertive, pioneering, competitive, courageous, selfish, headstrong, impulsive, foolhardy, angers quickly but doesn't bear grudges, athletic, likes danger and risk, leader, motivator. *Professions*: medicine, military, manufacturing, sports, carpentry, engineering. *Famous Arians*: Henry James, Marlon Brando, Bismarck, Joan Crawford, Charlie Chaplin.

Taurus, the Bull (20 April – 21 May) – loyal, stable, conservative, practical, patient, affectionate, good-natured, home-loving, sentimental, jealous, possessive, can erupt in anger, reliable, inflexible, committed, loves beauty and pleasure, aware of value of things, handles money well. *Professions*: banking, business, accounting, fashion, interior design, property management, singing, farming, architecture. *Famous Taurians*: Henry Fonda, Sigmund Freud, Shakespeare, Bing Crosby, Adolf Hitler.

Gemini, the Twins (22 May – 22 June) – quick-witted, changeable, talkative, versatile, crafty, mischievous, witty, clever, well-read, has something to say on everything, easily bored, may appear shallow and fickle. *Professions*: teaching, journalism, publishing, sales. *Famous Geminis*: Thomas Hardy, Marilyn Monroe, Duke of Edinburgh, Judy Garland, Arthur Conan Doyle, Marquis de Sade.

Cancer, the Crab (23 June – 22 July) – caring, emotional, sensitive, resistant to change, home-lover, fluctuating moods, artistic, good memory, sympathetic, caring, personable, easy to get on with, craves security, loves family, withdrawn, dislikes criticism, worrier. *Professions*: hospitality, cooking, catering, childcare, writing, property management, translating. *Famous Cancerians*: Rembrandt, Ringo Starr, Henry VIII, Gina Lollobrigida, Julius Caesar, Barbara Stanwyck.

Leo, the Lion (23 July – 22 August) – regal, self-centred, generous, warm-hearted, protective of those close to them and the weak, likes to be centre-stage, sensitive, likes praise and swayed by flattery, creative, dramatic, leader, likes elegance and class, nightlife, parties, games, gambling, believe they deserve the best, make big bold plans, look on the bright side. *Professions*: entertainment, beauty, cosmetics, gambling, speculative investing. *Famous Leos*: Napoleon, Princess Margaret, Mae West, Percy Bysshe Shelley, Alfred Hitchcock, Mussolini.

Virgo, the Virgin (23 August – 22 September) – practical, good communicator, shy, critical, concerned with health and hygiene, well-groomed, tidy, intelligent, hard-working, flexible, organiser, can be humble, perfectionist. *Professions*: nursing, service industry, health, nutrition, secretary, admin, teaching. *Famous Virgos*: Greta Garbo, Elizabeth I, Peter Sellers, Leonard Bernstein, D. H. Lawrence.

Libra, the Scales (23 September – 22 October) – diplomatic, refined, intelligent, thoughtful, sociable, warm, romantic, craves relationships, reasonable, loves comfort, luxury, strong sense of justice, aware of others' preferences, likes to lead but seeing all sides means decision-making difficult, peacemaker, desires balance and harmony, avoids confrontation. *Professions*: law, politics, arts, design, diplomacy, counselling. *Famous Librans*: Oscar Wilde, Julie Andrews, Nietzsche, Franz Liszt, Brigitte Bardot.

Scorpio, the Scorpion (23 October – 21 November) – energetic, passionate, deep, intuitive, secretive, self-controlled, wilful, stubborn, jealous, calculating, manipulative, cynical, sensitive, does not forgive easily, never forgets a slight, sees projects through despite obstacles, strong leader, incisive, motivated, enjoys financial security, enjoys danger. *Professions*: detective, forensic science, law enforcement, military, medicine, psychology, business. *Famous Scorpios*: Prince Charles, Marie Antoinette, Richard Burton, Charles de Gaulle, Pablo Picasso, Billy Graham.

Sagittarius, the Archer (22 November – 21 December) – fun-loving, friendly, philosophical, intellectual, straightforward, expansive, optimistic, naïve belief in good, lucky, generous, sharing, frank, blunt, honest, likes change, travel, fairly conventional, traditional, likes freedom of thought. *Professions*: higher education, law, medicine, import/export, publishing. *Famous Sagittarians*: Noel Coward, Winston Churchill, Frank Sinatra, Maria Callas, Walt Disney, Beethoven.

Capricorn, the Goat (22 December – 20 January) – responsible, disciplined, methodical, cautious, serious, pessimistic, works hard to attain things, aloof, shy, awkward, difficulty relaxing, can be lonely, respects power, authority and structure, traditional, ambitious, needs security, works hard to get rich. *Professions*: banking, government, mining, farming, construction. *Famous Capricorns*: Richard Nixon, Edgar Allen Poe, Loretta Young, Joan of Arc, Isaac Newton, Nat King Cole.

5. Zodiac quiz

Hold each sign up and ask the group to identify them. See if they can arrange them in the correct order.

6. See how many words can be made from: CONSTELLATIONS.

Week 4 – Royal Ascot

Equipment: flipchart, pens, paper, newspapers (for racing information), hats from charity shops or home to decorate (NB these can be reused for the Easter Bonnets and the Wedding activity in July), white material strips to make cravats for the gentlemen, and, if possible, top hats. *My Fair Lady* video (it has an excellent Ascot scene).

1. Reminiscence and discussion

Tell the group a little bit about the history of Royal Ascot: Queen Anne first saw the potential for a racecourse at Ascot in 1711 when she was out riding, she came upon an area of open heath not far from Windsor Castle and thought it was the ideal place for 'horses to gallop at full stretch'. The first meeting took place on 11 August 1711. The inaugural event was called

Her Majesty's Plate, worth 100 guineas – ask if the group can remember how much a guinea is worth (£1 and one shilling (1/-) or £1.05p). So 300 years ago it was a very good prize to compete for. The race was open to any horse, mare or gelding over the age of six, each carrying 12 stone. It was unlike the races we have today – all the horses were hunters, not the speedy thoroughbreds we are used to seeing. The race consisted of three separate heats of four miles, so the winner must have had enormous stamina. There is no record of the first winner.

The Gold Cup is the most famous race of the meeting, held on the third day, which is known as Ladies Day and attracts large crowds. This special race began in 1807 and with it started all the traditions of the Royal Enclosure.

Beau Brummell, a dandy and a close friend of the Prince Regent, decreed that men of elegance should wear waisted black coats, white cravats and pantaloons. Over the years this has evolved into the wearing of 'morning suits' and equally 'respectable' clothes for the ladies, who must wear hats. There was a Royal Stand in the 1790s, but the Royal Enclosure was built in 1845 when King George IV commissioned a two-storey stand. Entrance was by Royal invitation only.

In 1825 the Royal Procession began as an annual tradition, when the King and four carriages with the royal party drove up the centre of the course. The racecourse was run for the Sovereign by the Master of the Royal Buckhounds until 1901, when Lord Churchill became the HM Representative who ran the course and determined who entered the Royal Enclosure. In 1955 the rules of divorce were relaxed and divorcees were allowed to enter, but entry to the new Queen's Lawn was still governed by the court rules, so no divorcees were invited there! Nowadays everyone is welcome, but people have to apply in advance for the Royal Enclosure and new applicants must be sponsored by existing Royal Enclosure badgeholders (who have attended the Royal Meeting at least four times).

Ask the group if they can remember the most famous hat wearer, who wore fantastical hats designed by her son David. (Mrs Schilling.)

Ask the group if they know anything about the 'Sport of Kings', i.e. horseracing. Did they or their family follow the racing? Do they bet? Can anyone explain 'odds' – the price you get for your bet?

Do they prefer flat or 'over the sticks' (jump races)? Does the group know what the races with jumps are called? (Steeplechases – because in the olden days they were held on village streets and were run from one church steeple to another, jumping anything in their path. There are also hurdles races.)

2. Horse sense

Ask the group in general.

1. Does a horse lie down to sleep?...no
2. What is another name for a blacksmith who shoes horses?...farrier
3. Can a horse swim?...yes
4. What sex is the sire of a foal?...male

5. What does sire mean?...father
6. What are a horse's four different speeds of moving?...walk, trot, canter, gallop
7. What is a male foal up to three years old called?...colt
8. How can some experts tell the age of a horse?...by its teeth
9. What does a red ribbon in a horse's tail indicate?...it's a kicker!
10. How long does a horse spend grazing per day?...11–13 hours
11. In what are horses measured?...hands
12. How big is a hand?...4 inches (10cm)
13. Can a horse have feathers?...yes – the long hair on its ankles is known as 'feathers'.
14. What are the riders in a race called?...jockeys
15. The horse owners are recognised by...their colours
16. Even if they are old, the horse attendants are still...stable lads
17. Another name for a bookmaker...turf accountant
18. To put money on a horse...make a bet
19. Riding trousers are called...jodhpurs
20. ...and where did this word originate from?...India

3. Mad hatters

Give everyone a paper and pencil and ask them to design a 'wild' hat for Ascot. This could be played as Picture Consequences to take the pressure off the menfolk, with everyone drawing first the brim, then passing the drawings to the right. Everyone adds a crown to the brim, and passes to the right once more. Then ask everyone to add decoration, flowers, ribbons, birds, animal, etc. Show the finished hats around the group, one at a time. Using the hat collection, ask the ladies to select an Ascot hat in preparation for watching the race proper, or taking part in the[...]Cup Sweepstake (see next activity). Try and get the gentlemen to make a cravat each from the white material.

4. Sweepstake

Name the 'Cup' after your establishment, or make up another title.

On the flipchart make four columns: *owner – horse – colours – jockey.*

In the **owner** column write and number the names of all group members. Ask the group in turn to think of names for their horses – write the names in the **horse** column. Then ask them in turn for the colours they would like their jockey to wear and write those in the **colours** column. Then ask them to choose anyone they like to ride their horse – not necessarily a real jockey. The chart could look like this:

Owner	**Horse**	**Colours**	**Jockey**
1. Mrs Mary Smith	Sea Biscuit	purple and green	Elvis Presley
2. Mr Fred Jones	Neddy	red and yellow	Willie Carson

...and so on. For a bit of fun you could make one or two of the group aristocrats by calling them 'Sir' or 'Lady'.

On slips of paper write the number of each of the 'owners' and place them in a hat for a sweepstake. The group can put a sweet, a counter or 10p each in the kitty. Then invite another member of staff to draw out the 'winning number'. That 'owner' then takes the kitty.

On Lady Day, have a proper sweepstake – put the names of all the horses in the Queen's Cup in the hat and get the group to draw out one each for 10p. Then watch the race to see who is the winner of the kitty.

5. Straight from the horse's mouth

Ask the group to name a horse-related saying that fits the description.

1. Someone who shows an unsuspected accomplishment.

   A dark horse. This alludes to the trick of disguising a winning horse with dye and racing him.
2. Ask someone to be patient.

   Hold your horses. From slowing down a horse by pulling on the reins.
3. A famous quote from *Richard III* by William Shakespeare.

   A horse, a horse, my kingdom for a horse.
4. On the highest authority.

   Straight from the horse's mouth. Punters would ask the various racing stables for tips, and the hottest tips on who was likely to win were said to come from the horse.
5. Impossibility of coercing people into doing something.

   You can take a horse to water, but you can't make it drink. (Stan Laurel famously quipped, 'A horse may be coaxed to water...but a pencil must lead.')
6. Another matter entirely.

   A horse of a different colour.
7. To be practical, use your gumption.

   To have horse sense.
8. To go all out.

   Go hell for leather. From riding at speed using saddle, bridle and stirrups (all leather based).
9. Do not be rude enough to look for defects in a present.

   Don't look a gift horse in the mouth. Where its age, and therefore its value, can be ascertained.

10. Take control of a situation, quickly get on with the job.

    Take the bit between your teeth. When a horse does this, he is in control, not the rider.

11. Do things out of order.

    Put the cart before the horse.

12. Be superior, talk down to folk.

    Get on your high horse. This comes from the times when the aristocrats rode on the tallest, biggest horses and could talk down to the lower orders.

13. Be unable to rouse people from apathy.

    Flog a dead horse.

14. Put safety rules in place after an accident.

    Locking the stable door after the horse has bolted.

15. When we are getting older we are said to be like this.

    Long in the tooth. As a horse ages, its gums retract, making its teeth appear longer.

16. To stupidly change leaders in mid-project.

    Change horses in mid-race.

17. Begin a project again from the beginning.

    Start from scratch. Horse races used to start from a line scratched in the ground, so a false start meant they had to go back to the scratch.

18. Take a hint.

    A nod's as good as a wink to a blind horse.

6. Watch the video of *My Fair Lady* (or just the 'Ascot' scene).

7. See how many words can be made from: THE ROYAL ENCLOSURE.

Week 5 – Garden party

Over this week, plan for a garden party to be held at a weekend. Ask the group if they have been involved in garden parties/fetes. Have they any ideas for one? Discuss what, if any, the money raised is to be used for – this is a good advertising line and also gives the group a chance to discuss charity and good causes. It may be necessary to have a ballot to resolve the result, as there are so many worthy charities. It may be that the centre or home needs a specific piece of equipment, and having a fundraiser gives everyone 'ownership' of the equipment. Begin collecting well in advance for the tombola, bottle and cake/biscuit stalls. Often local shops and businesses are very generous with donations. The group and staff will (all being well) be generous with spare items such as bottles (any type of sauce, vinegar, oil, beer, etc.)

and unwanted gifts for the tombola, and homemade cakes/biscuits (or bought items, if Health and Safety do not allow homemade items).

Equipment required for each stall is listed under the relevant heading.

This activity is an opportunity for the whole group and their families/friends to participate in some way, however small – they also serve who only come and buy! Try to get the group to volunteer by designing a poster to advertise the garden party, assisting in running a stall or helping to set up.

Stalls

TOMBOLA

Table, prizes, books of raffle tickets, sellotape, tombola drum (one could be borrowed from the W.I., scout group or church; if not available, a large box will allow for ample mixing of tickets). Label items 1, 5 or 10 depending on odds for winning required, place all folded tickets in drum.

RAFFLE

Books of raffle tickets. Ask local companies and/or shops for prizes. Ask the oldest resident/client and the youngest staff member to draw the prizes.

GUESS THE WEIGHT OF THE CAKE

Ask a kind, good baker to make and weigh a cake, charge 25p a guess, and the winner has the cake.

HOW MANY BEANS IN THE JAR

Large glass jar, bags of jelly bean sweets or dried beans. Count out jelly beans or dried beans – a job for group members? Charge 25p a guess and the winner gets either the jar of jelly beans or a cash prize, dependent on how much raised by the stall.

BOTTLE STALL

Collect over time gifts of various bottles. Raffle tickets, container for raffle tickets. Number bottles for tombola.

HIT THE WHISKY BOTTLE WITH A £1 COIN

Bottle of whisky placed in centre of large piece of card/paper marked in one-inch squares. Ask people to throw/roll £1 coins at the whisky bottle, and write the names of those closest to the bottle in the square nearest to their coin. The person closest at the end of the fete wins the whisky, the rest forfeit their pounds!

CAKES, SCONES AND BISCUITS STALL

Donations from staff and clients.

GUESS THE NAME OF THE TEDDY BEAR/DOLL

People usually have a doll or teddy they are willing to donate. Ask the donor to give it a name. Keep a list of the names suggested, and charge 25p each name. The winner keeps the bear/doll.

FIND THE HIDDEN TREASURE

On a large piece of paper draw a desert island (complete with palm trees, rocks, cave, waterfalls and lake). NB a willing client could do this. Draw numbered squares all over the island. Choose which square hides the treasure (a box of chocolate/sweeties, or whatever). Sell the squares for 25p each, and the person who buys the chosen square wins the 'treasure' at the end of the fete.

PRIZE STRING

Various prizes. Lots of lengths of string, one of which is tied to a prize (bottle of wine/hankies/scarf/sweets, etc.). Tangle the strings and charge 25p–50p a go, depending on the value of prize. When you have 5–10 people each holding a string, ask them to pull and one *may* be tied to the prize, which the lucky person will keep. Set up after each 'win' until all the prizes are gone.

SPLAT THE RAT

Length of plastic drainpipe, length of strong string, tied to a furry piece of material and slotted through pipe, with the 'rat' visible at one end, a stick or wooden spoon. Someone with good reflexes is needed to pull the 'rat' through the pipe. Charge 25p a go for someone to see if they can hit the 'rat' with the stick or spoon before the stallholder pulls it back up the pipe. If they 'splat' the 'rat' they win £1.

BOWL AT THE SKITTLE

One plastic skittle (this could be made from a painted plastic bottle weighted with sand or water), three balls. Charge 5p for three balls (so that children are not priced out of the games). If you knock over the skittle, you win back your 5p.

FORTUNE-TELLER

You will need a volunteer who reads the tea leaves or cards and has a good knowledge of the clients. It is fun if they are willing to dress up as a gypsy fortune teller. Also required: a tent, booth or broom cupboard, with a table and two chairs.

FACE PAINTING

Children find this enjoyable. Perhaps a member of staff can do this.

NAIL PAINTING

Maybe a member of staff or a family member would volunteer for this.

TEAS

Tea, scones and jam or biscuits are a good moneyspinner.

Last-minute thoughts

- Wet-weather accommodation is essential in our usual summers.
- Local bands will come for a donation.
- Local dance groups will come for a donation.
- Icecream van may come and give a donation for the privilege.
- There may be a local Punch and Judy, clown or magician willing to appear.
- Ask a local dignitary/celebrity to officially open the fete. If none available, maybe the oldest resident/client would enjoy doing the honours.

Activities for July

Week 1 – A question of sport

Equipment: paper and pencils, flipchart and marker pen, slips of paper with different sports written on them, hat to put them into. Strips of ribbon, beanbags and numbered cards for target game.

1. Reminiscence and discussion

Ask the group about their school sports day. Did they have an annual Sports Day? What type of sports did they have? Did they have to participate in sport at school? What type of races did they have? Do they remember egg-and-spoon and sack races, relays and three-legged races? What sport did they enjoy the most? What excuses did they make up to avoid sport? At school did they have 'houses'? Can they remember the names and house colours of theirs? Did they have a school cup? a *Victor ludorum*? (This is an award for the champion of champions.) Has anyone played sports competitively? Has anyone been awarded a certificate for sport? What sports did they play when they were older? Does anyone still play a sport – e.g. bowls, darts or snooker? Has anyone got a funny story to share about playing sport? Do any family members play sport? Have they met any famous sportspeople? Did they know them as children? Can anyone swim? How did they learn? Did they learn at school? Did anyone play netball, football, hockey, lacrosse or do gymnastics? How have they changed over time – equipment, rules, attitude to refs, professional fouls, etc.?

Does everyone enjoy watching sport on TV? Which ones? Wimbledon? Snooker? Football? Motor racing? Horseracing, etc., etc.? Which football team do they support? Why? What do they think about footballers today, compared to when they were young? What sort of salaries did the old-time players get? What does the group think about David Beckham and the likes of Wayne Rooney? How do the ladies feel about sport? Do they find it boring? Which sports do they like best? List the choices of the men and women. How do they compare?

2. Sport 'Twenty Questions'

Write the names of different sports on slips of paper and put them in a hat. One member of the group chooses a slip and reads it, but must not show it to the group. The other group members each ask him/her a question in turn. The person with the slip of paper can only respond 'yes' or 'no'. The object of the game is to guess the name of the sport. Only 20 questions can be asked. The first person to guess the sport gets to choose another slip from the hat. If the sport is not guessed, the person with the slip of paper gets to choose again. The game ends when all the slips of paper have been taken.

3. Name that sport

(based on *More Mental Aerobics* page 81)

This quiz is played in teams, each named after a famous sports personality. Write down the answers, or take turns to answer.

1. 'Free-falling' is a sensation experienced in this sport...parachuting/bungee jumping
2. Climbing mountains is known as...mountaineering
3. Track and field events include these three basic body actions...running, jumping and throwing
4. A fibreglass pole is used in this sport...pole-vault
5. In this sport you get a tow from an aeroplane, a release, then, 'You're on your own'...gliding
6. If you use an epée, sabre or foil and wear a mask, what would you be doing?...fencing
7. A martial art from Japan which still uses Japanese terminology...judo
8. Name four throwing field events...discus, hammer, javelin, shotput
9. The Chinese are associated with this sport...table tennis, ping-pong
10. A shuttlecock is used in this sport...badminton
11. Unarmed combat using arms, legs, feet and head at incredible speed...karate
12. The most famous championships of this sport are held at Wimbledon...lawn tennis
13. The aim of this game is to put a round ball through a hoop...basketball/netball
14. You throw your opponent to the floor and hold him down for a count of 3...wrestling
15. The court for this high-speed game is an enclosed, four-walled area...squash
16. The 'Sport of Kings'...horseracing
17. British cavalry officers in India played this sport...polo
18. A bowler, fielders, batsman and four bases make up this game...rounders/baseball
19. 'Eagle', 'birdie' and 'tee' are terms used in this game...golf
20. This is also the name of an English public school...rugby
21. Riding a horse over jumps in a race...steeplechase

22. Horserace without fences…flat race
23. A wicket and a box are used in this game…cricket
24. National sport of Canada, played originally by North American Indians…lacrosse
25. A round stone, a brush and ice are needed to play this…curling
26. No ice, but skates for this sport…roller-skating
27. 'Bully off' and wooden sticks…hockey
28. You can play this on the beach if you have a raised net…volleyball
29. Can you paddle your own?…canoe
30. The sport of Robin Hood…archery
31. Dumb-bells, snatch and jerk are used in this sport…weightlifting
32. Two teams of eleven, one of whom can use his hands…football
33. You can use the horizontal bar, the floor or a horse for this…gymnastics
34. Oxford and Cambridge challenge each other annually at this…Boat Race/rowing
35. To wear the yellow jersey is a great honour…cycling (Tour de France)
36. Compulsory figures are completed in this sport…figure skating
37. Underwater ballet…synchronised swimming
38. 'Cleat', 'batten', 'tack' are terms in this sport…sailing
39. A small board on wheels is used by youngsters…skateboarding
40. A rucksack, map and strong boots…hiking
41. What sports are in a triathlon?…swimming, running and cycling
42. Small glass balls in a chalk ring…marbles
43. What game was featured in *Alice in Wonderland*?…croquet
44. 'Cue' and 'pot' are part of…snooker
45. Jumping over a series of these in a race…hurdles
46. Spectacular views from on high in a basket!…hot-air ballooning
47. An umpire is the official in…cricket
48. A corner coloured either red or blue…boxing
49. What happens in a velodrome…cycling
50. Nearly but not quite Union…Rugby League.

4. Sporty words

(based on *More Mental Aerobics*, page 143)

This can be played by two teams, named after football teams. Either read out the explanation and ask each in turn to *identify the term*, or read out the term and ask the team to give a *definition* and say with which sport it is connected.

Term with explanation	**Sport**
• *dribble* = passing football to oneself from one foot to other	football
• *Queensbury Rules* = ensure a safe and fair bout	boxing
• *half nelson* = a hold through opponent's armpit and round neck	wrestling
• *fairway* = mowed part of golf course between tee and green	golf
• *chequered flag* = signals end of race for a driver	motor-racing
• *cox* = steers boat and calls the stroke	rowing
• *axel* = free skating jump turning 1.5 times	figure skating
• *butterfly* = swimming stroke using both arms in a circular motion	swimming
• *LBW* = leg before wicket	cricket
• *caddie* = person who carries clubs	golf
• *hooker* = middle player who strikes for ball in scrum	rugby
• *tack* = go in zigzag course in sailing or all the saddles, harness etc., used in riding	sailing or riding
• *penalty spot* = area in front of goal where player gets to shoot at goal with only keeper defending	football
• *south paw* = boxer who leads with his left fist	boxing

Add more of your own sport words.

5. Sports quiz

Ask the group these questions in turn. Anyone in difficulty can be assisted by the rest of the group.

1. Which sport is associated with Wimbledon?...tennis
2. Which sport is associated with Lester Piggott?...horseracing
3. Who was The Greatest?...Muhammad Ali
4. Graham Hill was famous for...motor racing
5. What famous horse race is run at Aintree?...Grand National
6. How often are the Olympic Games held?...every four years
7. What has silly mid on, slips and gullies?...cricket
8. What does a caddie do?...carry golf clubs
9. How many players in a football team?...11
10. What equipment do you need to play badminton?...racket, net, shuttlecock
11. Who are the All Blacks?...New Zealand rugby team
12. In which sport do you use a 'cannon'?...billiards
13. Which sport has a Milk Race?...cycling
14. What happens at the White City Stadium?...dog racing
15. Who are the Gunners?...Arsenal FC
16. What do you use to make a cricket bat?...willow
17. How far do you run in a marathon?...26 miles
18. What is a chukka?...period of play in polo
19. Who plays for the Ashes?...England and Australia (cricket)
20. Who ran the first four-minute mile?...Roger Bannister
21. How many players in a Rugby Union side?...15
22. How many strokes under par is an eagle?...two
23. Which ball is potted after green in snooker?...brown
24. What is Bisley famous for?...shooting
25. What is the highest score with three darts?...180
26. Who won seven Olympic gold medals in 1972?...Mark Spitz
27. What is the penalty for refusing to jump?...3
28. When were the Rome Olympics held?...1960
29. Who was the most famous Victorian cricketer?...W. G. Grace
30. How long is a cricket pitch?...22 yards/20 metres
31. What race is from Putney to Mortlake?...the Boat Race
32. The person handling hounds in fox hunting is...a whipper-in
33. Who was the first man to win Wimbledon in three consecutive years?...Fred Perry
34. When was the football league founded?...1863
35. Can you name two sports with umpires?...cricket, netball, etc.
36. Can you name three sports with referees?...football, rugby, boxing

6. Football target game

In teams – each named after a football team.

Mark horizontal lines on the floor or ground with brightly coloured ribbons, each strip one foot wide and numbered 10, 20, 30, etc. In turn, each group member throws a beanbag to land on a strip between ribbons. The thrower is then asked a football question and if he/she answers correctly, the team scores the number on the strip – other team members can assist, facilitator can give extra clues.

7. Football quiz

1. Where is the FA Cup Final played?...Wembley Stadium
2. Name the Charlton brothers...Jack and Bobby
3. Name the two rival Glasgow football teams...Celtic and Rangers
4. How long is each half of extra time?...15 minutes
5. How many times do you have to score for a hat-trick?...three
6. Where does Pelé come from?...Brazil
7. How is play restarted when the ball goes over a touchline?...by a throw in
8. What colour are Manchester United shirts?...red
9. What is a foul?...an offence against an opponent
10. Who plays at Elland Road?...Leeds United
11. Who plays at Anfield?...Liverpool
12. Who is the only player who can handle the ball?...goalkeeper
13. Where is this allowed?...penalty area
14. Can you name the two clubs Brian Clough managed?...Derby County, Nottingham Forest
15. What was Bill Dean's nickname?...Dixie Dean
16. Who scored three goals in the 1966 World Cup Final?...Geoff Hurst

Add your own local football questions. A silver-paper World Cup could be presented to the winning team.

8. See how many words can be made from: A QUESTION OF SPORT.

Week 2 – Weddings

Preparation: staff to bring in own wedding dresses and photographs. (Ask clients in the week previous to bring in their wedding dresses and photos if possible.) Collect brides' magazines. using the internet, collect information on different cultures' wedding ceremonies, i.e. Islamic, Jewish, Sikh and Hindu wedding customs.

Equipment: flipchart, pens, paper. Information collected, photos and gowns, bouquet of paper/silk flowers. 'Wedding cake' (iced fruit cake).

1. Reminiscence and discussion

Ask everyone about their wedding, or a relative's or friend's if their own is not appropriate. Can everyone remember where they were when they were proposed to, or proposed? Ask the ladies how were they asked and what they replied, and the gentlemen how they asked and what was reply. Did they have to get permission from the father of their love? Was it intimidating? Do the youngsters do this today? How long was the engagement? What was their engagement ring like? Do they still have it? Can they still wear it today? Did they choose it or was it part of the proposal and a surprise to them? Did anyone receive a ring that was a family ring, an heirloom? Did they have a hen or a stag night? What did they do? What does the group think about the kind of stag and hen nights of today – costs and destinations?

Who helped organise the wedding? Where did they get married? What did they wear? Can anyone remember how much their wedding suit/dress cost? Can they still get into it today? (This is also one for the staff to answer if they have brought their gowns in.) Compare them to today's prices. Does anyone remember Princess Diana's dress? (A picture would be ideal.) Did anyone make their own outfit? How many bridesmaids did they have? What colour were their dresses? Has anyone been a bridesmaid? What did they wear? People can hire wedding outfits today. Did that happen when they were getting married? Who was Best Man? Has anyone been a Best Man? What was his speech like? Where did they have the reception? What food did they have? What was their cake like? How many tiers? Talk about the wartime rationing and how they used a cardboard fake cake cover over a spongecake, family and friends saving food coupons to buy ingredients for the cake. What flowers did they have? Discuss the language of flowers. (See internet for info: type 'Language of flowers' into search engine.)

Did they wear a veil or a hat? Who gave them away? Was it a church or a civil ceremony? What music did they have? Can anyone remember their vows? Do they like today's vows? Do they feel they are more relevant if they are composed by the people involved? Would anyone like to remake their vows, or even make different ones now? Should women still promise to 'love, honour and *obey*'? What do they feel about prenuptial agreements? Does this devalue commitment or is it a wise thing to do in the present climate? What do they think about the high divorce rate today, compared to when they were young?

Pass around any pictures you have of different ceremonies.

Talk about any local wedding traditions they may know of, and their meanings, for example, sweeps, throwing rice, confetti or coins, being carried over lychgates.

2. Budget for a wedding

In small groups, get clients to estimate the cost of a wedding, allowing for:

- wedding dress
- four bridesmaids' dresses
- photographer
- reception at a smallish venue

- groom's outfit
- Best Man's outfit
- flowers
- cars
- cake.

Compare each group's costs and then inform them of current prices.

3. The Wedding Breakfast

Have 'wedding cake' and a cup of tea and show photos and dresses to clients. Discuss wedding customs regarding wedding cake, confetti, shoes, bouquet, flowers, bridesmaids, choosing the date, dress, 'something old, something new', crossing the threshold, the honeymoon. Information can be obtained from website www.weddings.co.uk/info/tradsupe.htm

Was anyone tempted to elope?

4. Famous couples

(based on *Mental Aerobics* page 28)

On the flipchart list the group's suggestions. Some starters:

- Mrs Simpson and Edward VIII
- Solomon and Sheba
- Richard Burton and Elizabeth Taylor
- Antony and Cleopatra
- Posh and Becks
- Romeo and Juliet
- Margaret and Denis Thatcher
- Winston and Clementine
- Mickey and Minnie Mouse
- Nancy and Ronald Reagan
- Richard and Judy
- Charles and Camilla
- Debbie McGee and Paul Daniels
- Queen Elizabeth and the Duke of Edinburgh
- Tony and Cherie Blair

5. Toss the bridal bouquet

The 'bride' (a member of staff) stands or sits in front of the group and throws a bouquet of paper/silk flowers to a group member, for him/her to catch, the person who catches the bouquet then becomes the 'bride' and throws it to the next person, and so on. This game improves hand/eye coordination and concentration, and is fun.

6. See how many words can be made from: WEDDING CAKE.

Week 3 – Holidays and honeymoons

Equipment: travel brochures, flipchart, pens, copies of picture puzzle on page 142 and picture message on page 143.

1. Reminiscence and discussion

Ask if everyone went on honeymoon after their wedding (to tie in with last week's activities). Where did they go and for how long? Could people afford to go abroad then? Does anyone have a funny or embarrassing honeymoon story? What destination would they choose now as their dream honeymoon? Where is the most romantic place they can think of?

What is their earliest memory of seeing the sea? How old were they? Who were they with? What is the first holiday they can recall? How old were they? Who took them away? Where did they stay and how did they get there? Coach? Train? Car? Bicycle? What in particular has stayed with them all this time? Where did people go on holiday when they were young? Did they go on school trips or Sunday school outings? Where did they go? When they were first married with young children, could they afford holidays? To where? How many weeks paid holiday were they entitled to, compared to today's workers? How did they save up for holidays – did they have a savings club? Could people afford a holiday every year? Where was their favourite destination? Did anyone go to Butlins, Pontins or any other holiday camps? Did they enter the competitions? Is there a Glamorous Grandma or a Knobbly Knees Champ amongst them? Can anyone remember any famous Red Coats? Has anyone been camping? Stayed on a barge? In a caravan? Rented a holiday cottage? Holiday Camp? Was *Hi-de-Hi!* true to life?

Did anyone wear hats with a funny logo, e.g., 'Kiss me quick?' What is the funniest souvenir they have given or received? What would people class as a typical holiday souvenir?

Has anyone been abroad? What is the most beautiful tourist destination? Is anyone planning a holiday this year? Where? Where would they like to visit if they could? Look at travel brochures, discuss the cost of travel, carbon footprint...

2. All at sea

(based on *More Mental Aerobics* page 74)

In two teams named after holiday destinations. Ask teams to write down the answers and exchange answer sheets for marking at the end of the quiz.

1. Found in the ocean and in the bath...a sponge
2. This has five or more pointed arms...starfish
3. The tentacles of these creatures make them look like flowers...sea anemones
4. The sea teems with this basic food source of many sea animals...plankton
5. What does the famous Irish folksong cry?...'Cockles and mussels, alive, alive-oh!'
6. Who lives in others' shells?...hermit crab

7. Someone who studies shells is a...conchologist
8. Transparent and often stinging...jellyfish
9. They cling to the ship's bottom...barnacles
10. A shell shaped like a Chinese hat...limpet
11. Blue in the water, red on the plate...lobster
12. This creature is covered in prickles...sea urchin
13. A shell shaped like a fan...scallop
14. The largest mammals...whales
15. These animals live together in a reef...coral
16. How is a pearl made?...from a grain of sand in an oyster
17. Lots of fish swim in...shoals
18. This birds likes rubbish dumps and shores...gull
19. A cocktail can be made from these...prawns
20. How does an octopus protect itself?...squirts ink
21. The ebb and flow of water...tides
22. What did whalers cry when they spotted a whale?...'Thar she blows!'
23. Which nationals like their fish raw?...Japanese
24. The male of this fish carries the young...seahorse
25. These flatfish can become enormous...rays
26. The name in literature of the great white whale?...Moby Dick
27. What is a seasoned sailor called?...a Sea Dog
28. When can he have a drink?...when the sun is over the yard arm
29. What would he drink?...rum
30. Who was the pirate captain in *Treasure Island*?...Long John Silver

3. Where in the world?

(based on *More Mental Aerobics* page 235)

Still in teams – ask in turn. If a team is unable to answer a question, give it to the opposing team. Where would you see or experience the following?

1. Beefeaters, ravens, Crown Jewels?...London
2. Whisky, bagpipes, tartan?...Scotland
3. Hot climate, Taj Mahal, crowds?...India
4. Cuckoo clock, skis, Heidi?...Switzerland
5. Pyramids, camels, sand?...Egypt
6. Opera House, outback, corks on hats?...Australia

7. Clogs, tulips, windmills?...Holland
8. Cigars, Che Guevara, samba?...Cuba
9. Tea Ceremony, paper houses, kimonos?...Japan
10. A tower with a tilt?...Pisa
11. Table Mountain, Mandela, gold?...South Africa
12. Guinness, Giant's Causeway, Blarney Stone?...Ireland
13. Sausages, Bier, leather shorts?...Germany
14. A canal and a special hat?...Panama
15. Birthplace of the Olympics and Plato?...Greece
16. Was British until 1997, an island, horse racing?...Hong Kong
17. The Andes, beef, Evita?...Argentina
18. Voodoo, Port-au-Prince, Caribbean?...Haiti
19. Elegant women, fashion, Eiffel tower?...Paris
20. Castanets, flamenco, straw donkeys?...Spain
21. Cricket, pudding, moors where you should wear a hat?...Yorkshire
22. Nuts, there's a lot of coffee?...Brazil
23. Krakow, birthplace of Chopin?...Poland
24. Daffodils, leeks, rugby?...Wales
25. Island in the Mediterranean, Turks and Greeks share it?...Cyprus
26. The first Disneyland, Keys, Orlando?...Florida
27. Kibbutz, the Wailing Wall?...Israel
28. Victoria Falls, elephants, was Rhodesia?...Zimbabwe
29. Wine, croissants, cuisine?...France
30. Battle of the Flowers, thick cream?...Jersey

4. 'I packed my suitcase' – memory game

Clients seated in a circle, allow the person with the poorest memory to go first. Make the statement, 'I am going on a trip. I will pack in my suitcase (select something beginning with letter A, maybe 'Aspirin')'. The next person says, 'I will pack Aspirin and (they select something beginning with B)', and so on. The object is to see how many things can be remembered. Assistance can be given by facilitators, but preferably by group members.

5. What's wrong with this holiday resort?

Give everyone a copy of the picture on page 142.

Answers: boy digging with spade handle, sand pie wrong way up from tipped bucket, no supporting strut to deckchair, woman knitting with wooden spoons and she has one trouser leg and one shoe on, her companion has only one darkened lens, steps missing, 'To the Beach' sign pointing wrong way, car wheel missing, door on first floor of building, lighthouse shines in land and is visible in day time, fishing rod missing, mast at end of rowing boat on beach, man swimming in bowler hat, sea gull has missing wing, only one oar in rowing boat, billowy clouds have level tops, smoke blowing in opposite direction to flag on ship, wave patterns differ, child riding donkey backwards

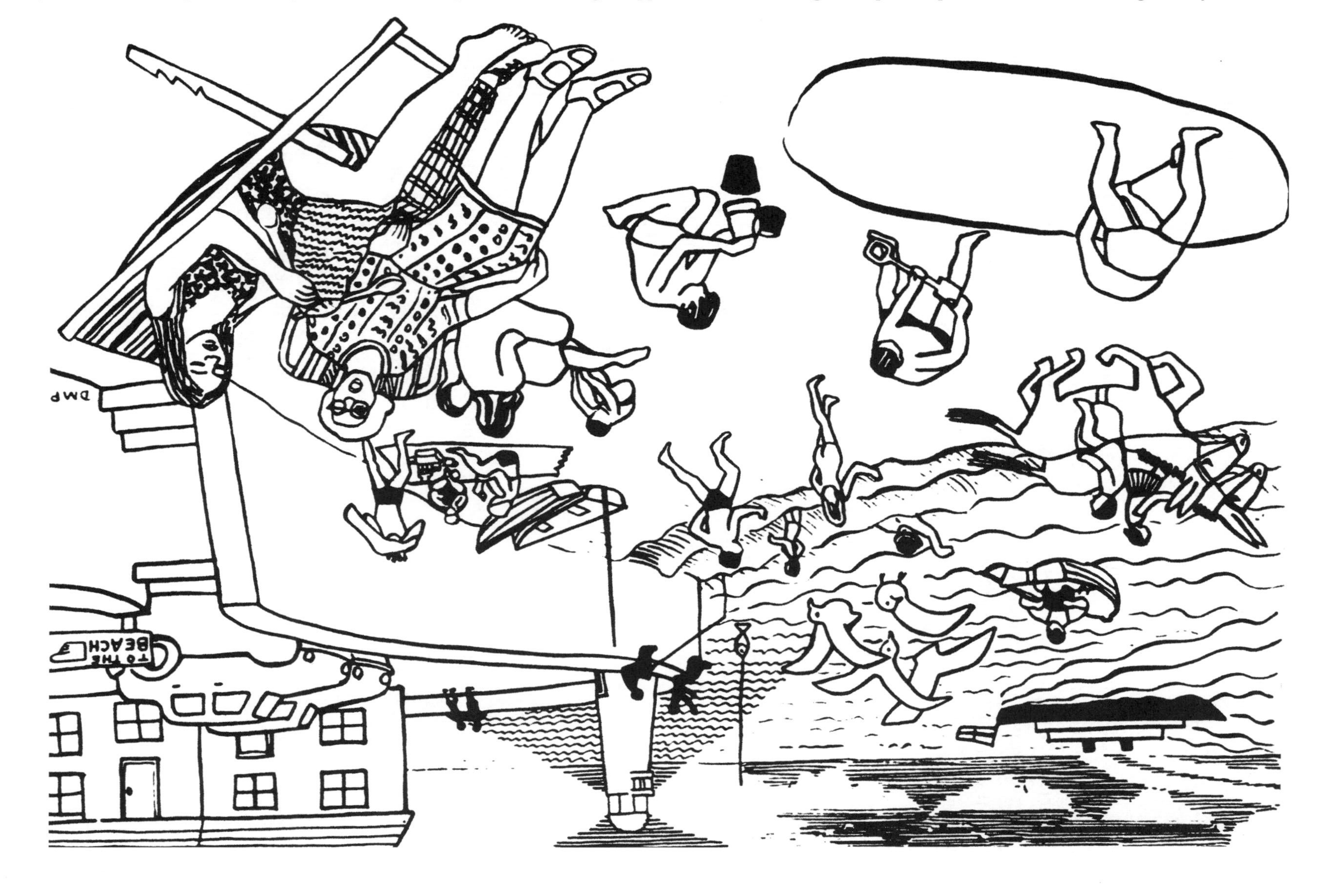

6. Holiday 'Hangman'

Use words associated with holidays and destinations, for example: 'sandcastle', 'bucket and spade', 'airport', 'caravan park', 'suncream', etc.

7. Picture message

Can group members decipher it?

PICNIC PICTURE STORY

On Friday as the
was shining we made some
and put some in
a and drove the to
the . We found a
and caught a with a .
We climbed a and ate our
and picked some Then
we walked through the
and sat on a and saw a
. We watched the
set, and went home in
the .

Answer: As the sun was shining we made some sandwiches , put some coffee in a flask and drove the car to the country .We found a lake and caught a fish with a rod. We climbed a hill and ate our picnic and picked some flowers. Then we walked through a wood and sat on a log and saw a bird. We watched the sun set and went home in the car.

8. Feely bag

Place different holiday items in a beach bag and pass it round the group for identification by just feeling the objects – for example: sunglasses, lolly stick, tube of suncream, sandals, passport, spade, bus ticket, toilet bag, novel, sunhat, camera, etc.

9. See how many words can be made from: BLACKPOOL.

Week 4 – Local traditions

Equipment: flipchart, quiz questions, playing cards (large size if possible), carpet bowls. Word search grid (page 145). Pencils. Prepared tray of different objects for Kim's Game. This week's activity will require research in your area for any customs and traditions specific to the locality. Library and local news offices plus internet are useful for this. Local Quiz questions.

1. Reminiscence and discussion

Discuss your local traditions, ask about participation, show any historical pictures you may have to stimulate memories. Pass around any pictures of the traditional activity. Does anyone recognise people in the pictures? Ask if anyone or their families/friends have taken part in them? Can anyone recognise the streets or shops in the photos? Discuss how your locality has changed. Can they remember old shops/buildings that are no longer there? Ask what sort of things they did in the past to prepare/take part in the tradition. Any funny happenings? Do they know the origins of the custom? Do they think the young people will continue to keep these traditions going? Was there a carnival procession or a street party in their area? Was there rivalry between different areas or streets?

If possible, recreate a part of your local tradition. For example, in Derbyshire a well-dressing could be constructed by the centre.

2. To maintain a local carnival atmosphere, play carpet bowls in teams named after streets in your area.

3. 'Play your cards right'

Continuing friendly rivalry, still in teams, play this game, using large playing cards and questions from 'Trivial Pursuit' or any quiz book.

4. Kim's Game

Put objects associated with your local area on a tray. Let everyone look at and touch the objects on the tray, then remove the tray from sight. Ask how many objects can be remembered and write them on a flipchart. Bring the tray back to check how many are correct. Remove the tray from sight, remove one object and see who notices what has been removed. Repeat for a few times.

5. Quiz on your local town

Street names, shops past and present, location of schools, churches, pubs, local heroes and dignitaries, any famous people born there – make up suitable questions.

6. See how many words can be made from the name of your county, or main town, if the county name is too short. Example: YORKSHIRE.

7. Word search

Give each person a copy of the grid, with names of your famous local buildings, products and people hidden in the squares.

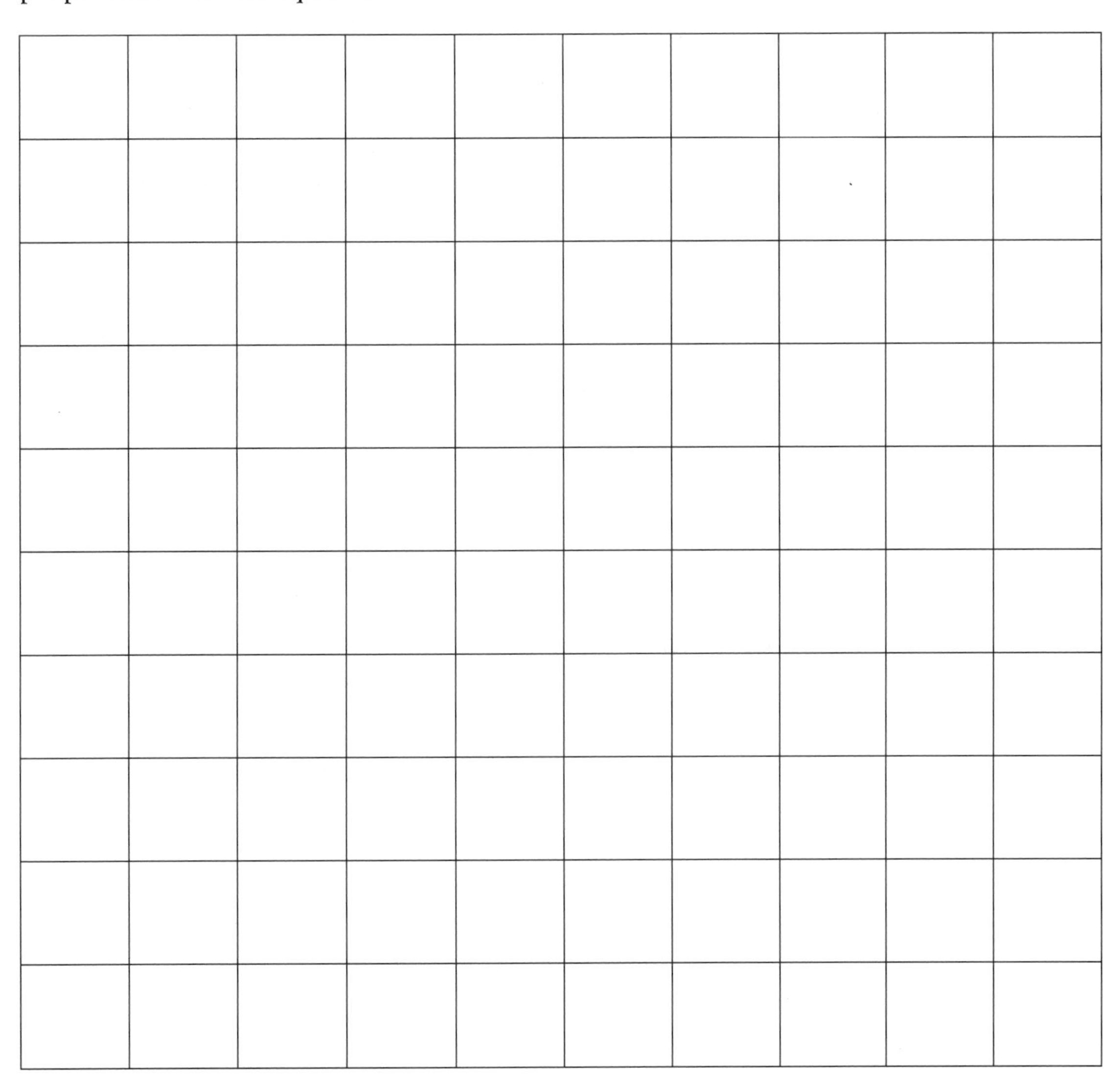

Can you find the following words in the grid above?

Activities for August

Week 1 – Food, glorious food

Equipment: collect pictures of old-fashioned cooking utensils. Copies of the word search (page 150) and 'teapots' quiz (page 154) for each person, flipchart, pens and pencils. This is a very full section, so spread out the quizzes over a few days.

1. Reminiscence and discussion

Talk about the food they enjoyed when they were young. Did their mother have a baking day? Which day was it? Did they help? What sort of things were made? Did they bake when they were first married? What happened in rationing during the War and just after? Could they still get all the ingredients for baking or did they have to substitute certain things? Can anyone remember any of the strange recipes, e.g. Wooton Pie, and what was in them? Do they think people were fitter then? Why do they think people are getting obese today?

Do they think food tastes as good today? If not, why? Do they eat less than they used to? Did the men of the house used to be served first? Why was that? (Usually because they had a hard, physical job with long hours and would be very hungry, or simply because they were the head of the family.) Did they always have enough to eat when they were young? Did they sit around a table to eat? Do they still do that now at home? Do they still bake? If so, what do they make? Can the men bake? Do they cook for themselves? Any disasters? How did they manage if they were left to cope? Does anyone have meals delivered? What are they like?

What do they think of the ready meals and cakes we buy today? What is everyone's favourite cake? biscuit? hot meal? And their most favourite meal of all? (Under headings, make lists on the flipchart.) Is the group mainly sweet-toothed? Is that a recent preference, or because after the shortage of sugar in their early days, they can now indulge their sweet tooth? How many different types of biscuits can they name? Does everyone use the same recipe for pastry?

What cookery books can they remember? Do they still have them – perhaps could bring them in to show the group? Can they name any famous cooks past and present? What TV cookery programmes can they name? Who is their favourite TV cook? Does anyone ever actually try the recipes they see on TV, or do they watch, then have a ready meal? Does anyone collect recipes from magazines, newspapers or friends? What do they think about food scares? Are they affected by them? Was food in the olden days fresher? cleaner? more tasty? What do they think about all the vast choices and variety we have these days? What about the over-packaging of foodstuffs – cellophane-wrapped bananas, wrapped turnips and coconuts?

2. Ten-minute challenges

(based on *More Mental Aerobics* page 183)

In teams of three or four named after TV cooks, each to have paper and pencil and one person to write the answers.

a) List *things to do with food preparation* in the past and now. Allow 10 minutes per section.

   The past: (for example) butter churn, paddles, mortar and pestle, mincer, eggwhisk, wooden spoon, rolling pin, grater, solid fuel range/Aga cooker, copper pans, meat safe, isinglass egg preserver, muslin to strain fruit, lemon squeezer.

   Now: (for example) fridge, freezer, electric/gas cooker, single featured and combi microwaves, breadmaker, icecream maker, food processor, juicer, electric mixer, non-stick pans, wok, garlic press.

b) List as many *pies* as they can – for example, lemon meringue, Mississippi mud, pork, apple, gooseberry, blackberry and apple, bannoffee, fly pie, steak and kidney.

c) List *terms of endearment* that are food-based – for example, sugar plum, sweetiepie, cupcake, honey, sweet pea, treacle tart, honey bun, candy kiss.

Score ten points for the most in each category. The second team gets eight points, third gets six points, and so on.

3. Food quiz

Still in teams, have one person to write the answers and at end of quiz swap papers for marking.

1. Juice from beets and canes make this...sugar
2. Named after a German city and eaten at a BBQ...hamburger
3. A very popular bird, who can be cowardly...chicken
4. A bubbly celebration drink...champagne
5. Stringlike pasta...spaghetti
6. Scotland's favourite little biscuit...shortbread
7. Goes well with roast beef...Yorkshire pudding
8. Italian food that can be delivered to the door...pizza
9. Fishy starter with pink sauce...prawn cocktail

10. Can't make a sandwich without this...bread
11. Tossed on Shrove Tuesday...pancakes
12. What meanz Heinz?...beanz(s)
13. What do we call cooked icecream?...baked Alaska
14. Dry roasted, roasted or in a shell...peanuts
15. Where would you be served 'borscht'?...Russia
16. What is served at a continental breakfast?...croissants
17. Eaten on Burns Night...haggis
18. What is a Devon cream tea?...scones, butter, clotted cream and jam
19. White cabbage, carrot, onion and salad cream?...coleslaw
20. How do we eat icecream without a dish?...cornet, wafer, on a stick or in a choc bar
21. Sugary, greasy ring...doughnut
22. Popular at parties in the sixties – cheese or chocolate...fondue
23. Salad invented in famous American hotel...Waldorf
24. Chased in a children's story...Gingerbread Man
25. Goes with lamb...mint sauce
26. The nation's favourite cuppa...tea
27. What was drunk in the sixties coffee bars...frothy coffee
28. Harry Ramsden cooked these...fish 'n' chips
29. Gary Lineker advertised what?...Walker's crisps

4. From the menu

Still in teams.

1. Not from the set menu...à la carte
2. Melted cheese on toast...Welsh Rarebit
3. Beaten egg, fried in special pan with cheese, etc...omelette
4. Little toasted or fried squares of bread...croutons
5. Cooked fish and potatoes covered in breadcrumbs...fishcake
6. Little squares of filled pasta...ravioli
7. Tall glass of icecream, fruit and sauce...Knickerbocker Glory
8. A starter of meat or fish paste...pâté
9. Stew topped with potatoes...Lancashire hotpot
10. A wobbly, fruity dessert...jelly
11. A very expensive fungus...truffle
12. Steak cooked in a pastry case...Beef Wellington
13. A preserve on toast for breakfast...marmalade

14. How many different ways can a potato be served?...Mashed, roast, chipped, baked, crisps, rosti
15. Very small fish in oil...anchovies
16. Children loved this milky dish shaped in a mould...blancmange
17. Some are not strong enough to knock the skin off...rice pudding
18. Fried leftover potatoes and cabbage...bubble and squeak
19. Chocolate cake from a large German wood...Black Forest gateau
20. Mashed potato on beef/lamb mince...cottage/shepherd's pie

Add more of your own.

5. Foody sayings

(based on *More Mental Aerobics* page 119)

Ask the group in general.

1. If you drop the ball...butterfingers
2. Round and fat...butterball
3. Easy or simple...piece of cake
4. Go crazy...go bananas
5. A good-hearted person...salt of the earth
6. Admit you are wrong...eat humble pie
7. Other things to do...other fish to fry
8. A tricky situation...bit of a pickle
9. Comfortable and prosperous place...land of milk and honey
10. Everything is great...peachy
11. After a failed romance we are told...there are lots more fish in the sea
12. Sweet person...honey
13. Give someone their comeuppance...cook their goose
14. When too many people are involved...too many cooks
15. To cap it all...take the cake, biscuit
16. Dismiss an idea...throw cold water on it
17. Look smug...like a cat who's got the cream
18. A lovely person...a sweetiepie
19. Justify doing something harsh to accomplish a goal...can't make an omelette without breaking eggs
20. A beautiful complexion...peaches and cream

Ask the group if they can think of any more.

6. Find the vegetables

D	A	N	D	E	L	I	O	N	F	E	N	N	E	L
R	S	A	L	S	I	F	Y	R	O	C	I	H	J	N
A	U	B	E	R	G	I	N	E	O	K	R	A	E	A
H	T	R	U	F	F	L	E	S	S	E	R	C	R	E
C	I	L	U	O	M	U	S	H	R	O	O	M	U	B
M	A	R	R	O	W	S	W	E	D	E	B	P	S	H
O	P	T	A	R	T	U	R	N	I	P	E	A	A	C
N	E	O	D	P	O	T	A	T	O	L	E	R	L	N
I	P	M	I	C	A	B	B	A	G	E	T	S	E	E
O	P	A	S	P	R	O	U	T	S	N	R	N	M	R
N	E	T	H	C	A	N	I	P	S	G	O	I	A	F
B	R	O	C	C	O	L	I	P	E	A	O	P	R	A
I	S	B	R	O	A	D	B	E	A	N	T	K	T	S
C	A	U	L	I	F	L	O	W	E	R	C	O	I	P
E	C	R	E	S	S	E	C	A	L	E	A	H	C	A
L	K	I	D	N	E	Y	B	E	A	N	R	L	H	R
E	A	C	O	U	R	G	E	T	T	E	R	E	O	A
R	L	E	E	K	G	R	E	E	N	S	O	P	K	G
Y	E	L	E	T	T	U	C	E	O	I	T	A	E	U
S	C	A	R	L	E	T	R	U	N	N	E	R	S	S

Can you find the following vegetables?

DANDELION, FENNEL, SALSIFY, AUBERGINE, OKRA, TRUFFLES, MUSHROOM, MARROW, SWEDE, TURNIP, POTATO, CABBAGE, SPROUT, BROCCOLI, PEA, CAULIFLOWER, CRESS, CALE, BROAD BEAN, KIDNEY BEAN, COURGETTE, LEEK, LETTUCE, SCARLET RUNNERS, GREENS, PEPPER, TOMATO, FRENCH BEAN, CELERY, ASPARAGUS, CARROT, BEETROOT, PARSNIP, ARTICHOKE

7. Fruit and veg

Ask each person to identify the fruit or veg.

1. A type of brandy, on top of iced bun, on a cocktail stick…cherry
2. Throw things at me at fairs, I feed the birds…coconut
3. We are a 'peel' of bells in St Clements…oranges and lemons
4. Tread on me or give me to the sick…grapes
5. Bright red, grown on canes, or a rude noise…raspberry
6. Fuzzy skin but so sweet with cream…peach
7. Green and one of three…gooseberry
8. English ones taste best, red, grow in beds and smell of summer…strawberry
9. Exotic, have many black seeds and a wrinkled skin…passion fruit
10. Can't get a straight one, skin can be dangerous…banana
11. Grown in orchards and makes scrumpy…apples
12. With 11 to make Cockney stairs…pears
13. Make a boat for a starter…melon
14. Grow in hedgerows, great in pies with apples…blackberry
15. Twins are said to be like us when we are in our shells…peas
16. Embarrassing root vegetable with red, staining juice…beetroot
17. My curds look like a brain…cauliflower
18. A shortage of me caused Ireland's troubles, mash me with bangers…potatoes
19. French, red, kidney, broad *and* baked…beans
20. I bring tears to your eyes…onion
21. I help with night vision…carrot
22. Welsh emblem…leek
22. Halloween is my best time…pumpkin
23. Good as soup or sauce and in salads…tomato
24. With tatties on Burns' Night…turnip (neeps)
25. Not as green as I'm – looking!…cabbage

Add more of your own or ask the group to make some up.

8. Cookery quiz

1. Why do we sometimes beat steak?…to tenderise it
2. What is a bouquet garni?…a bunch of herbs in a stew
3. Why don't strawberries freeze well?…high water content
4. What is deer meat called?…venison
5. What is shortening?…fat used in pastry making

6. What does basting mean?...ladling melted fat over roasting meat
7. Which wine is served at room temperature?...red
8. Which cheese is served with spaghetti bolognaise?...Parmesan
9. What is the handling of bread dough called?...kneading
10. What are smoked herrings called?...kippers
11. Where are marmalade oranges from?...Seville
12. What are croutons served with?...soup and salad
13. What are Red Windsor and brie?...cheeses
14. What helps jam set?...pectin
15. What is the strongest flavoured member of the onion family?...garlic

9. Food quiz 2

Ask the group as a whole:

1. Which far northern city is famous for its fruitcake topped with almonds?...Dundee
2. A famous pudding from Derbyshire...Bakewell
3. Scottish biscuit for cheese...oatcake
4. What are Pontefract cakes made from?...liquorice
5. A pudding sometimes eaten for a first course...Yorkshire
6. A Royal who burnt the cakes...King Alfred
7. The Geordies eat 'singing hinnies'. What are they?...griddle cakes
8. Made for lead miners with savoury and sweet fillings in one pastry case...Cornish pasties
9. French flan with cheesy custard filling...quiche lorraine
10. Lancashire sugared, flaky pastry filled with currants...Eccles cake
11. An amphibian in batter...toad in the hole
12. Choux pastry finger filled with cream covered in chocolate...eclair
13. A Queen of cakes...Victoria sponge
14. We are no longer allowed to put silver three penny bits in this!...Christmas pudding
15. A boozy break...brandy snap
16. Pink and plain sponge squares covered in marzipan...Battenburg
17. Often in tiers and cut with ceremonial knife...wedding cake
18. A favourite of the man who watches the flock...shepherd's pie
19. One a penny, two a penny, or an angry rabbit!...hot cross bun
20. A green and stupid dessert...gooseberry fool

Add more of your own.

10. Easy cookery quiz

1. Which fruit is squeezed?...lemon
2. What is served with lamb?...mint sauce
3. What are jacket potatoes?...potatoes baked in their skins
4. Shallots and chives are in which family?...onion
5. Where are frog's legs eaten?...France
6. In what do you pickle onions?...vinegar
7. Which meat accompanies Yorkshire pudding?...roast beef
8. How do you thicken cream?...whip it
9. What do you serve apple sauce with?...roast pork
10. What is the essential ingredient in an omelette?...egg

11. Everything stops for tea!

Give a copy of the teapots picture on page 154 to each person. Ask them to find the matching pairs.

12. See how many words can be made from: INGREDIENTS.

NB Inform everyone that the theme for next week is 'Antiques' and ask staff and clients to bring in a 'treasure' from home.

Week 2 – Antiques

Equipment: using sales catalogues, laminate different pictures of antiques and beside each give a small description and a selection of prices, including the real value, to use in Valuation quiz. Reminiscence box. (Over time, put together items from the past – rag dolls, wooden pegs, toys, pots, thimbles, sock mushroom, butter pats, etc., to make a reminiscence box.) Auction room picture (page 157) for each client. Word search (page 158) either on flipchart or photocopy. The week before, ask staff or clients to bring in any special treasure they may like to share. Flipchart and pens.

1. Reminiscence and discussion

Talk about antiques, does anyone collect them? Ask if anyone has any antiques at home that have been passed down through the generations. Can anyone think of things their parents or grandparents used that are now antiques? Stone hot-water bottle, shaped copper and pot jelly-moulds, shaving mugs, jam pans, log boxes, warming pans, cameras, lamps, etc. Has anyone still got any furniture that once belonged to their grandparents?

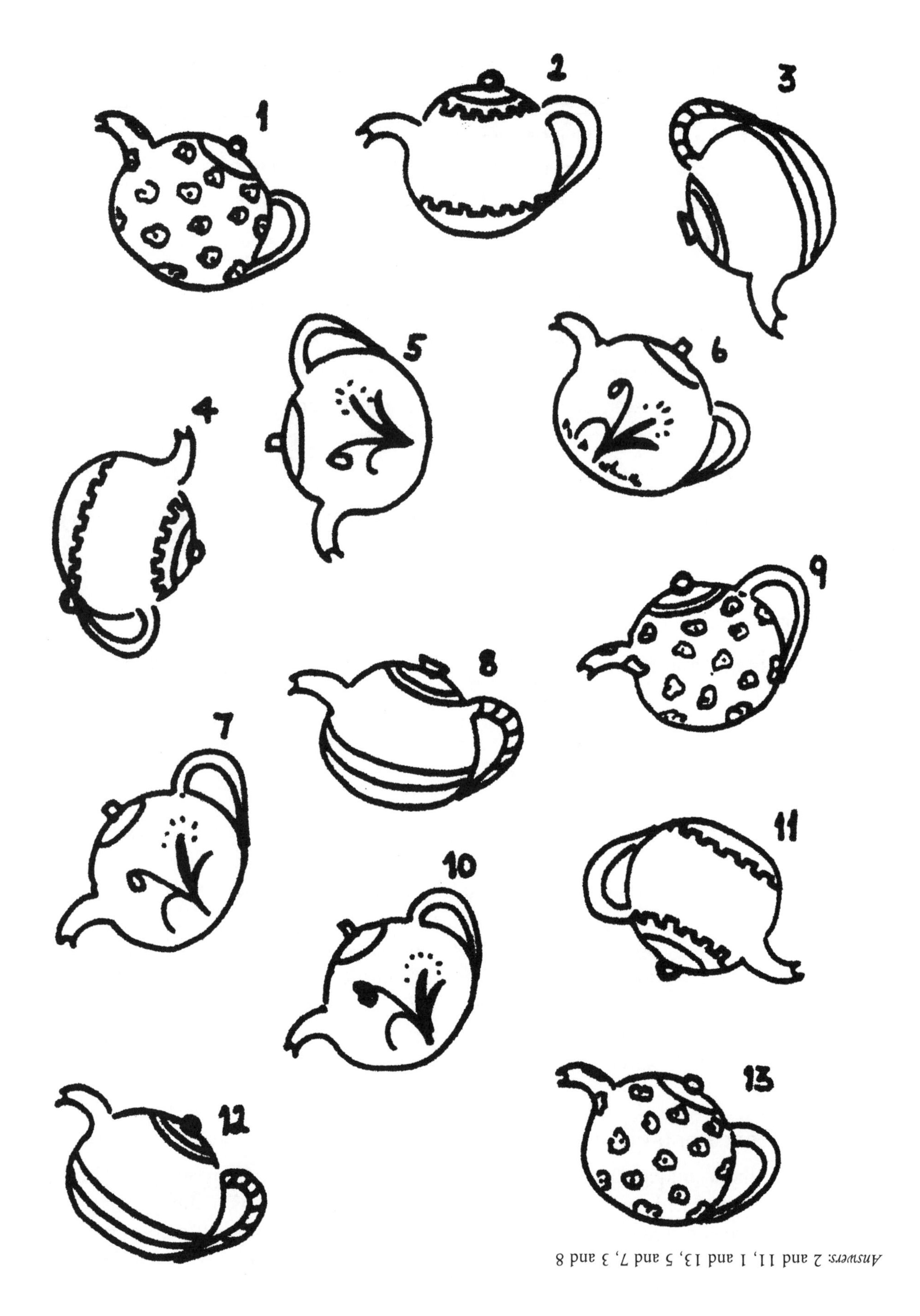

Answers: 2 and 11, 1 and 13, 5 and 7, 3 and 8

Does anyone have a collection of anything? China? Glass? Snuff boxes? Coins? Stamps, Books? Do they think the younger generation will appreciate them? Has anyone seen anything on TV antiques programmes they can remember having in their childhood home? Can they believe the valuation of these things nowadays? Can anyone make a guess at what the next collectable items will be? Has anyone begun a collection of possible value? Does anyone watch the antiques programmes on TV? Can anyone tell if the participants are disappointed in the valuations? Do they enjoy the surprise when people are given a good unexpected price? Which antiques programmes on TV can they name? (*Flog It, Going for a Song, Antiques Roadshow, Bargain Hunt, Boot Sale Challenge, Cash in your Attic?*)

Can anyone remember the name given to the furniture available in the War? 'Utility' – why was it called this? Did anyone have to buy it? Is it still going strong?

2. Antiques display

Show all the items brought in, ask what they are used for. Why is this special to the owner, how old is it, do they have a value for it, either monetary or sentimental? Are there any special ways of caring for antique goods that people could share with the group?

If you have a reminiscence box, display some of the objects on a table, ask the group to look at the objects for a minute or so, then, in turn, to select one object that brings back a memory for them. When all have chosen something, ask each of them to share their memory with the group. For example, many may have fond – or not – memories of wearing darned socks, or darning socks, if there happens to be a sock mushroom on show.

3. Valuation quiz

In teams named after a TV antiques show. Pass round the laminated pictures and ask teams to write down their estimated value. When all have seen all the pictures, show them in turn and hold a mock auction (volunteer auctioneer required) before giving the real auction price.

4. 'Antiques Roadshow' quiz

As a large group.

1. How long has the show been on TV?...since 1979
2. Who is the new presenter?...Fiona Bruce
3. Who was the first presenter?...Arthur Negus
4. Followed by...Hugh Scully
5. There was a female presenter who also read the news...Angela Rippon
6. What furniture could have a balloon back?...chair
7. How do you date silver?...by its hallmark
8. EPNS stands for...electroplated nickel silver
9. When was the Georgian period?...the period covering the four King Georges, 1714–1830

10. When did Queen Victoria reign?...1837–1901
11. Art Nouveau is an artistic movement. True or false?...true
12. Where do you send items for sale?...auction house
13. Can you name a famous one?...Christie's/Sotheby's
14. What is the famous blue-and-white Chinese china?...Willow Pattern
15. What make of china is this?...Spode
16. Can you name another famous blue-and-white china?...Wedgwood
17. Can you name the famous teddy-bear manufacturer?...Steiff
18. How would you recognise one?...he has a button in his ear
19. What defines an 'antique'...something over 100yrs old
20. What do you need to prove a picture is not fake?...provenance

5. Using the flipchart, list as many words as possible to describe something 'antique' or 'old'.

Examples:
bygone, old, rarity, heirloom, curio, ancient, veteran, vintage, classic, outdated, old-fashioned, obsolete, museum piece, curiosity, worn, patina, relic, antiquarian, archaic, retro.

6. Anti-'QUE' words

(from *Mental Aerobics* page 108)

Using the flipchart to record their answers, ask everyone to list as many words as they can with '-que' in them – for example:

quench, queen, quell, queen, quest, bequest, Quebec, bequeath, request, inquest, querulous, oblique, parquet, deliquent, sequel, squelch, squeak, consequence, racquet, cheque, pique, bouquet, clique, torque, Jacqueline, croquet, Mozambique, tourniquet, queue, sequence, etiquette, boutique, squeal, squeeze, question, queasy, squeamish, aqueduct, plaque, basque.

7. The auction room

Give each client a copy of the picture on page 157 and, using the flipchart to write down the answers, ask the group:

- how many chairs can they find and what different types are they?
- how many tables and their different functions?
- how many beds? Is the chaise longue counted as a bed?
- how many clocks?

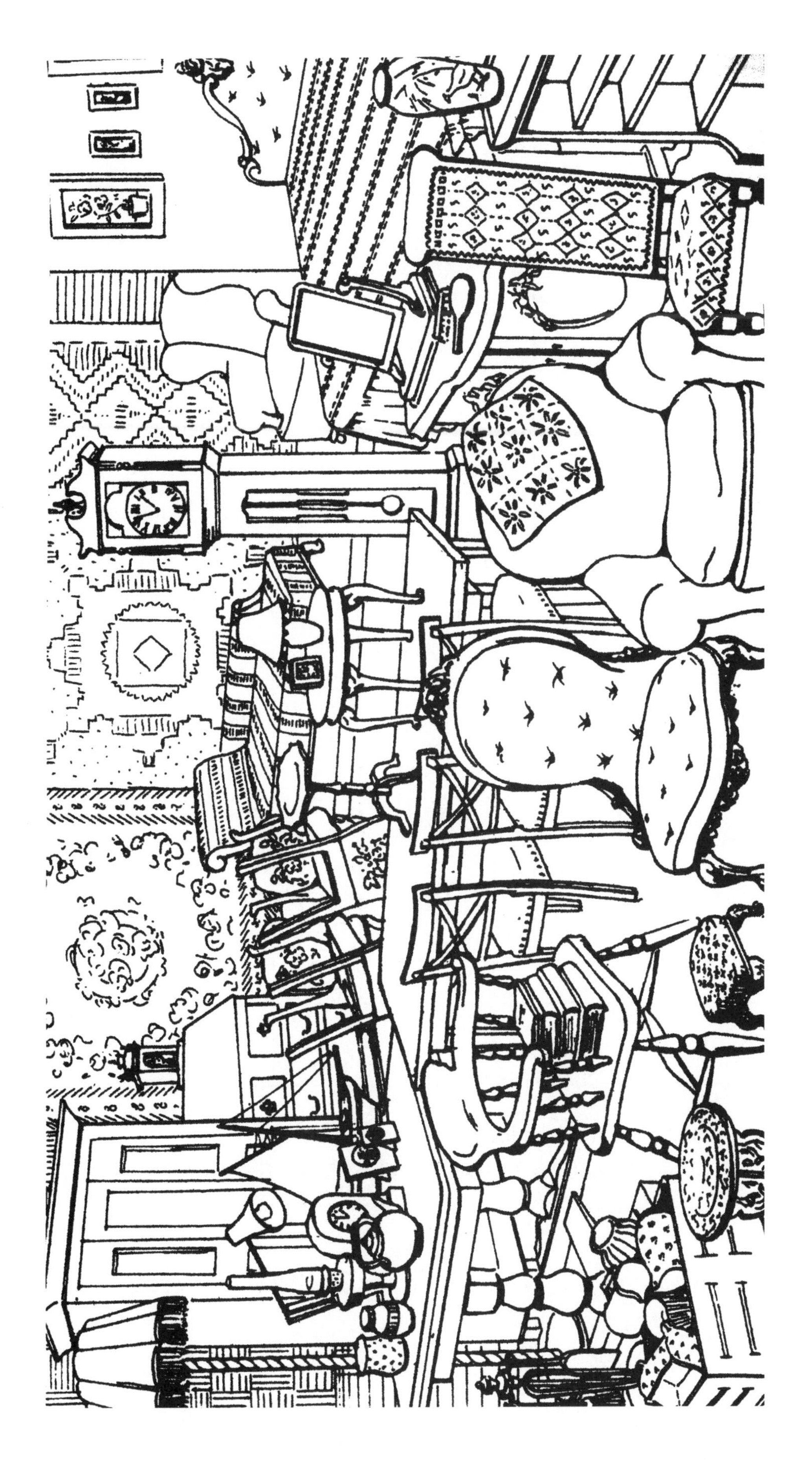

List all the objects they can name in the picture. Do they have anything like these objects at home? Has anyone ever been to an auction? What did they buy? Was it nerve-racking bidding? Did they overspend?

8. Word search

B	T	U	Y	G	F	A	W	O	D
U	A	E	K	C	P	M	R	N	E
M	B	C	A	C	H	L	I	R	C
F	L	Z	N	D	G	A	T	I	A
D	E	Y	I	C	L	F	I	S	N
O	S	A	H	E	A	G	N	R	T
B	E	D	C	U	S	G	G	S	E
O	L	R	B	L	S	W	A	G	R
C	O	M	M	O	D	E	S	U	P
P	M	O	V	W	A	A	C	J	H

Can you find these words hidden in the grid?

PORCELAIN, CHINA, CHAIR, GLASS, JUGS, DECANTER, DAY BED, WRITING TABLES, COMMODES

9. See how many words can be made from: GOING FOR A SONG.

10. See how many words can be made from: ANTIQUES ROADSHOW.

Week 3 – pubs and inns

Equipment: flipchart, quizzes, any pub-type games equipment available. A pub quiz and pub games are included in the session. Each day, feature a different pub game. Over time it is a good idea to collect copies of any pub quizzes you may take part in, and various pieces of equipment for pub games, e.g. darts, dominoes.

1. Reminiscence and discussion

Talk about the 'local'. Did everyone use a public house when young, or was it just for the menfolk? Can they remember fetching a jug of ale for their father from the local pub? Was there a special window for youngsters to do this? What was the legal age to be served with alcohol in a bar? Can they remember the cost? Is the pub still there? What were the opening hours? Did the pub open on a Sunday? Has anyone owned or worked in a pub? What is everyone's favourite drink? Do they go into pubs now? For a drink or a meal? Has the atmosphere changed in pubs from when they were young?

Did anyone play for the darts, dominoes or quiz team? Do any pubs still have special areas to play tabletop skittles, cribbage, darts, cards or dominoes?

Did families go into pubs? Were meals served? Was there ever a 'lock in'? Has anyone got any funny stories of youthful exploits? Stag nights? Any fundraising activities held by their local pub?

Using the flipchart, list the names and localities of the pubs in your area. Have any changed their names or signs? Can anyone remember any funny pub names they may have seen – on holiday or nearby? How the Wetherspoon Group became so named stems from the story of the founder being told by a teacher that he would never amount to anything, so he determined to prove him wrong and have his name in every town he could. He began in a small way, offering a different style of pub without juke boxes, child-friendly, with cheap and cheerful food and a quiet atmosphere. Didn't he do well!

What do they think of the current extended opening hours and the drunken behaviour of some youngsters? What can we do to encourage more responsible drinking? Are the pubs better for the smoking ban?

2. Drinks round memory game

The first person names a drink, the person next to them repeats it and adds one of their own...and so on, as far as possible without repeating a drink. Assistance can be given by rest of the group if memory is faltering.

3. Pub signs

On the flipchart make a list of pub names. Ask (include staff in this) for any strange ones such as The Frog and Nightgown, The Waltzing Weasel, The Blazing Rag. Did anyone collect beer mats? A beer mat collector is called a 'tegestologist'!

4. Pub games

In teams named after pubs, play a different game each day. Give an explanation of the game's origins.

1. DARTS

A target game where small, weighted, arrow-like missiles are thrown at a round, numbered board. The boards were originally made from cork, compressed paper or elm wood. Today they are made from sisal and are known as 'bristle' boards. Darts developed from archery and was played on miniature archery targets. The game became popular in public houses in the mid-nineteenth century but became formally organised only in the 1920s. In 1924 representatives of the licensed trade, some major breweries, dart board manufacturers and the staff of the *Morning Advertiser* met in London to set up the first darts league in public houses and to formulate the rules. The game has become more and more popular with the advent of televised World Championships, and is the most popular pub game for both men and women. The line the players throw from is called the 'oche', supposedly derived either from the use of the brewers Hockey and Sons' beer crates to measure the distance – so you were said to be 'toeing the hockey' – or from an old Flemish word meaning 'notch', or from Old English *hocken* meaning 'to spit', i.e. the throwing distance was as far from the board as you could spit!

2. DOMINOES

Played by two or more people with 28 small, flat, rectangular blocks originally made from ivory or bone, but now made from wood or plastic. The game originated in China and was introduced into Europe in the mid-eighteenth century. A very popular game in pubs and clubs. A variation is 'Fives and Threes' where the object of the game is to get the end two 'bones' (slang term for dominoes) to add up to a sum divisible by 5 or 3 to give a score.

3. BILLIARDS

A table game for two or more players, using balls and cues. English billiards is played on a table with pockets, and carom (French) billiards on a table without pockets. The earliest mention of billiards is in 1429 in France, and it is thought to be related to such games as shuffleboard and croquet. Louis XI of France had a table and Mary Queen of Scots complained when she was held captive that her table had been removed. A reference in *Antony and Cleopatra* (1609) to them playing billiards is considered to be Shakespeare's sly joke. The first World Professional Championships were held in 1870.

4. SNOOKER

A game usually for two players, derived from billiards using the pocketed table, cues and 22 balls. The game was invented in 1875 at the Ooty Club in Southern India by British Army officers. Colonel Sir Neville Bowes Chamberlain invented the game and gave it the name of 'snooker', a slang word for clumsy army cadets. In 1885 John Roberts brought the game back to England. The John Roberts Billiards Supply Company commercialised the game with sales of snooker sets. The first professional game was held in 1927. The televised championships became extremely popular with the advent of coloured television – especially amongst the older ladies!

5. DRAUGHTS

A chequered board game similar to chess, using simple counters rather than pieces, but with the same objective: to take as many of the opponent's pieces as possible, or else immobilise them so they can't make a move. It originated in Europe in the twelfth century, probably in France. In the early game capture of pieces was optional, but in 1535 a compulsory capture rule was introduced in France. The game was taken by English settlers to Northern America.

6. BINGO

Many pubs now have organised bingo games. The object of the game is to mark off the numbers on a previously numbered card as they are randomly selected from a thick material bag containing 100 numbered discs. The first to fill a card shouts 'House', as bingo was called 'housey housey' in England. It was also known as 'Lotto' in the 1880s. It may have been derived from a seventeenth-century Italian game called *Tumbule.*

7. BAGATELLE

A popular game in southern pubs, it has many variations, with the object of plunging balls into cups sunk into a wooden board six to ten feet long, with the holes at the farthest point from the players. Origins are sketchy, but may have some link with marbles or nine-men-morris.

8. BAR SKITTLES

Can be shaped like mushrooms or thin posts. Usually in the pub version the ball used to knock them down is attached to a post by a string – a much safer option than allowing folk to throw objects in an enclosed space – and the skittles are attached to a board with strings. (If skittles are not available they can be improvised using plastic bottles weighted with sand or water.)

9. CARD GAMES

Cribbage is the only card game that can legally be played for money in English pubs. It requires a long scoreboard with pegs, probably based on the ones used by the Ancient Egyptians. The players move their pegs up the outside and down the inside of the board, with the front peg showing the current score and the rear one the previous score.

Whist is one of the oldest card games, first referred to in 1529. It probably derived from the sixteenth-century game of 'English game trump'. There have been many changes in the game, some of which evolved into bridge.

Pontoon is a card game with the object of scoring 21 or as near as possible. Everyone is dealt two cards, then gets more cards by 'twisting' and tries to 'stick' without 'busting' as they play against a 'banker'.

10. BACKGAMMON

The oldest of all pub games, which came to England in the eleventh century, probably brought back by the Crusaders. It quickly became popular in the taverns as a chance to gamble and, in spite of laws passed to stamp it out, has continued to flourish to the present day.

5. Pub quizzes

Still in 'pub' teams, do the quiz of the day. It may be a good idea to run the quizzes like a pub quiz with teams of four or five. Have one person writing the answers and everyone in the team contributing. After ten questions exchange papers with another team and get them to mark, keep a running total of scores.

PUB QUIZ 1

1. Name the building that holds books for borrowing...library
2. If children play truant what do they do?...stay off school
3. Which bird is often called Polly?...parrot
4. What animal was the hero of *Watership Down*?...rabbit
5. What do Americans call the boot of a car?...trunk
6. What reference book would you use for spelling?...dictionary
7. What is a fortified wine and also a kind of harbour?...port
8. Who ate curds and whey?...Little Miss Muffet
9. What is the past tense of steal?...stole
10. What is the plural of wolf?...wolves
11. Who went through the looking glass?...Alice
12. What is the title of the book about Mowgli?...*The Jungle Book*
13. What is the word for a book written by someone a) about their own life? and b) about another person's life?...a) autobiography b) biography

14. What does the Latin phrase *bona fide* mean?…'in good faith'
15. Who is the hero of J. K. Rowling's books?…Harry Potter
16. What does ESP stand for?…extrasensory perception
17. What are two collective nouns for a group of whales?…school or pod
18. What two words can you get from a floor covering?…car and pet
19. What does OHMS stand for?…On Her Majesty's Service
20. Who lives in a pride?…lions
21. Which town is associated with Shakespeare?…Stratford-upon-Avon
22. If you 'chance your arm' what do you do?…take a risk
23. Who wrote *The Shining*, *Rose Madder* and *Misery*?…Stephen King
24. What means 'to hobble' and is also floppy?…limp
25. Is a coracle a council meeting place, a prophet or a boat?…boat

PUB QUIZ 2

1. What word is a boy's name, a duck's beak and an invoice?…Bill
2. While the King was counting out his money, what was the Queen doing?…eating bread and honey
3. Which short word can be placed after feather, sick and flower?…bed
4. What is the collective noun for a group of crows?…a murder
5. What does NSPCC stand for?…National Society for the Prevention of Cruelty to Children
6. Who wrote the longest-running West End play, and what was it called?…Agatha Christie; *The Mouse Trap*
7. What does UN stand for?…United Nations
8. What does Delia Smith write about?…cookery
9. Who did Fagin and the Artful Dodger take under their wing?…Oliver Twist
10. What does an adjective do?…describes a noun, e.g. *red* book
11. What does RSPB stand for?…Royal Society for the Protection of Birds
12. Who wrote *Bleak House*?…Charles Dickens
13. What reference book lists words with similar meanings?…thesaurus
14. Which of the Brontë sisters wrote *Wuthering Heights*?…Emily
15. What does TUC stand for?…Trades Union Congress
16. Is a braggart a petty criminal, a part of a horse or a boastful person?…a boastful person
17. Who wrote *The Canterbury Tales*?…Chaucer
18. Who was Sherlock Holmes' evil enemy?…Moriarty
19. What means a fruit, to age and an assignation?…date

20. What do the initials QC mean?...Queen's Counsel
21. Whose World War II diaries gave us an insight on religious persecution?...Anne Frank
22. In the horror story, who was shipwrecked off Whitby?...Count Dracula
23. If you have 'short arms and deep pockets' what are you?...mean or unwilling to spend your money
24. Which Norse god was Thursday named after?...Thor
25. A golf course at the seaside and parts of a chain...links

PUB QUIZ 3

1. What does PTO stand for?...please turn over
2. How many people speak in a monologue?...one
3. If you are 'tickled pink' how do you feel?...happy, really pleased
4. What are the letters of the alphabet that are not vowels?...consonants
5. Was it George Orwell or George Eliot who wrote *The Road to Wigan Pier*?...George Orwell
6. Who is Agatha Christie's lady detective?...Miss Jane Marple
7. Which newspaper had the nickname 'The Thunderer'?...*The Times*
8. Who wrote *Great Expectations*?...Charles Dickens
9. What is the paper cover on hardback books called?...dust jacket or jacket
10. What is the collective noun for a group of kangaroos?...a troop
11. In English grammar past, present and future are all what?...tenses
12. What book is Louisa May Alcott best-known for writing?...*Little Women*
13. Who is the national poet of Scotland?...Robbie Burns
14. What is the plural of sheep?...sheep
15. Is a minuet a gun, a dance or a type of castle tower?...dance
16. What is a collective noun for hens?...flock or brood
17. What is a pseudonym?...a name other than your real one, usually used by authors
18. Which word describes a person going red with embarrassment?...blush
19. Which word means to illustrate and also to tie in a contest?...draw
20. Which author had her book *Pride and Prejudice* rejected by a number of publishers?...Jane Austen
21. Who was the Belgian detective with little grey cells?...Hercule Poirot
22. What would you be if you are 'long in the tooth'?...elderly
23. Which prolific author wrote 26 books in one year?...Barbara Cartland
24. What does 'absence' make?...'the heart grow fonder'
25. What is sci-fi short for?...science fiction

PUB QUIZ 4

1. What is the collective noun for a group of dancers?...a troupe
2. What does MW stand for on a radio?...Medium Wave
3. Who robbed from the rich and gave to the poor?...Robin Hood
4. Did he live in Epping Forest, the New Forest or Sherwood Forest?...Sherwood Forest
5. What is the past tense of eat?...ate
6. Who wrote *The Sherlock Holmes Mysteries*?...Sir Arthur Conan Doyle
7. Which ancient Greek fell in love with himself?...Narcissus
8. Which animal is the book *Ring of Bright Water* about?...otter
9. What do Americans call cloakrooms?...restrooms
10. Who wrote *Sense and Sensibility*?...Jane Austen
11. Is a barnacle a type of oar, a shellfish or an ancient weapon?...shellfish
12. Who was Dr Jekyll's evil persona?...Mr Hyde
13. If you 'bend over backwards' what do you do?...try very hard to please
14. What is a mortician?...an American undertaker
15. Complete the title of the play *Two Gentlemen of...Verona*
16. What was the name of the horse in Anna Sewell's book?...Black Beauty
17. Who sold his cow for a handful of beans?...Jack (and the Beanstalk)
18. How many days did it take Phileas Fogg to go round the world?...80
19. If you 'burn the candle at both ends' what are you doing?...overworking
20. Which word means both attractive and 'quite'?...pretty
21. What do Americans call autumn?...fall
22. Which of Shakespeare's plays brings actors bad luck?...*Macbeth*
23. If you are a 'stick in the mud' what are you?...resistant to change
24. But if you 'turn over a new leaf', you will do what?...make a fresh start
25. In which book does Wendy Darling look after the Lost Boys?...*Peter Pan*

PUB QUIZ 5

1. In which pantomime does Widow Twanky appear?...*Aladdin*
2. What does UFO stand for?...Unidentified Flying Object
3. Who was the peg-legged pirate in *Treasure Island*?...Long John Silver
4. What did Ben Gunn long for on his desert island?...a little bit of cheese
5. What is a writing instrument and a holding area for sheep?...pen
6. If you 'spilled the beans' what would you do?...reveal the truth
7. Which sport did Dick Francis write about?...horseracing

8. What was the novel about a great white whale, written by Herman Melville?...*Moby Dick*
9. Where are the Inspector Morse stories set?...Oxford
10. Complete the play title *Antony and*...*Cleopatra*
11. Who according to the Old Testament was the oldest man who ever lived?...Methuselah
12. Who wrote *A Tale of Two Cities*?...Charles Dickens
13. What attribute does Tuesday's child have?...full of grace
14. Who saw a 'host of golden daffodils'?...William Wordsworth
15. Hemingway set the novel *For Whom the Bell Tolls* in which war?...the Spanish Civil War
16. A word that means elevator and to raise something....lift
17. Yorick appears in which Shakespearean play?...*Hamlet*
18. What was King Arthur's sword called?...Excalibur
19. Is cartography the study of oceans, volcano watching, or map-making?...map-making
20. Which country has pyramids and pharaohs?...Egypt
21. Which country's flag has a red maple leaf on it?...Canada
22. Which country's flag has a white cross on a red background?...Switzerland
23. Which city has the Golden Gate Bridge?...San Francisco
24. What is the capital of Australia?...Canberra
25. Is Auckland in New Zealand's North or South Island?...North

Week 4 – Soaps

People with memory difficulties may need more prompting because the soaps are mostly recent events and may not be part of their long-term memory process, but they may still be an enjoyable part of their day.

Equipment: flipchart, pens, prepared soap character quiz – collect pictures of soap stars and laminate them, with relevant questions attached. (*Examples of questions*: What soap is he/she from? What is their character called? Who is their partner? What job do they do? Is there any distinguishing feature to his character – such as Roy's carrier bag, etc.? Any major event in their character's life? Are they famous in another type of entertainment, as Barbara Windsor was? Remember to supply the answers!) Tape signature tunes from the soaps. Copies of the word search (page 170) for each person.

1. Reminiscence and discussion

Using the flipchart, make a list of the soaps clients watch, to see which are the most popular. Does anyone listen to *The Archers*? Can they hum the signature tune? Remind them how Billy Connolly thought this was a better tune than the official National Anthem.

Ask if the soaps are as good today as they used to be. Can they remember any of the soaps which are no longer broadcast today? – Include the radio ones such as *Mrs Dale's Diary*. Does anyone know why these programmes are called 'soaps'? (Because in the USA soap manufacturers sponsored these daily shows about the lives of a set of people.) Who are their favourite characters and why? How close to real life do they think soaps are? Point out the anomalies, such as how lax the work practices are, everyone going to the café for breakfast, being in the pub all the time, how everyone uses the launderette instead of a washing machine.

How do they feel about the newspapers filling their pages with soap gossip as if it was real? Are they annoyed when they reveal the future story lines? Do they remember when JR was killed, and was that the start of the newspapers' obsession with soaps? Do they remember the advertisers sponsoring the soaps? Can anyone remember the first adverts we had? ('You'll wonder where the yellow went...? The Esso sign means...? Murray mints, Murray mints, the too good to...? A Mars a day...? Hands that do dishes...? Ahhhhh...? Someone's mum just doesn't know...?') Do they remember the Oxo Family? The Gold Blend love story? the dashing man in black with the Milk Tray? The PG Tips chimpanzees? Do they think today's adverts are too arty? Can they understand them?

What are the clients' favourite programmes, other than soaps? Quizzes? Cookery? Antiques? Chat shows?

What do people think about Oprah and the people who go on such reality shows? Have programmes improved since the fifties, sixties? Is there too much explicit violence/sex these days? Which do they think is the worst influence on young children? Should they watch TV unsupervised?

2. Soap characters and signature tunes quizzes

In teams. Use the materials that you have prepared for these quizzes. A different quiz can be done each day

3. Soap trivia quizzes

Update these as and when. Still in teams.

CORONATION STREET QUIZ

1. Who was the Rovers' first landlady?...Annie Walker
2. Who looked after the Mission and wore a hairnet?...Ena Sharples
3. Who had three flying ducks on their wall?...Hilda and Stan Ogden
4. What was Stan's job?...windowcleaner
5. What was Elsie Tanner's son called?...Dennis

6. Who did Deirdre first work for?...Len Fairclough
7. Who was Ken Barlow's uncle?...Albert Tacklock
8. Who was Ena Sharples' friend?...Minnie Caldwell
9. Who used to run the Corner Shop?...Alf Roberts
10. Who is the only original cast member?...William Roache (Ken Barlow)
11. Who had a GI as one of her husbands?...Elsie Tanner
12. Who owned the factory and what did he make?...Mike Baldwin, underwear
13. Who was Annie Walker's barmaid?...Bet Lynch
14. What is Betty's favourite dish at the Rovers?...hotpot
15. Who married Alf Roberts?...Audrey
16. What is her daughter's name?...Gail
17. How did Emilie Bishop's husband die?...he was shot
18. Who is Toyah's stepfather?...Les Battersby
19. Who runs the café and what is it called?...Roy Cropper runs Roy's Rolls
20. Who owns the garage?...Kevin

EASTENDERS QUIZ

1. Who is Lisa's mother-in-law?...Pauline Fowler
2. Who is Phil's brother?...Grant Mitchell
3. Who plays his mother?...Barbara Windsor
4. What is the pub called?...The Queen Vic
5. Who were the landlords?...Angie and Den Watts
6. What was their daughter called?...Sharon
7. What was Dot Cotton's son called?...Nick
8. What job did Arthur Fowler do?...market cleaner, gardener
9. Who did the job when he died?...Robbie
10. What was the old doctor called?...Dr Legg
11. Who looked after the launderette?...Pauline and Dot
12. Who owned the launderette?...Mr Popadopulos
13. How many sons has Pauline Fowler?...two
14. Where is Michelle living now?...America
15. What illness did Mark have?...he was HIV positive
16. Who shot Phil Mitchell?...Lisa
17. Which family has five daughters?...the Slaters
18. What is Mark's brother called?...Martin
19. Who is Pauline's nephew?...Ian Beale
20. Which famous river is shown on the street map?...the Thames

EMMERDALE QUIZ

1. What is the name of the pub?...The Woolpack
2. Who was the first landlord?...Amos Brierley
3. Who killed Christopher Tait's father?...Kim Tait
4. What is the name of the notorious family?...Dingal
5. What are the vets called?...Zoe Tait and Paddy
6. Who is the vicar?...Ashley
7. Who became the Mayor and Mayoress?...Eric and Gloria Pollard
8. What is the name of Christopher's business?...Tait Haulage
9. Which two disasters killed off a few villagers?...a plane and bus crash
10. What did Seth do before retirement?...he was a gamekeeper
11. How did Jack Sugden's last wife die?...in a fire
12. When Emmerdale first started, who was the principal family?...the Sugdens
13. What were Jack's mother and brother called?...Annie and Joe
14. Who is the Irish character?...Ray
15. What is Seth Armstrong's partner called?...Betty
16. Who is his girlfriend and where does she work?...Louise, part owner of the pub
17. Who runs the Post Office?...Mrs Hope
18. Has Chris Tait always been wheelchair-bound?...no, only since the plane crash.
19. Who is Trisha's godfather?...Alan Turner
20. What was Terry's occupation before he came to Emmerdale?...professional Rugby player and landlord

SOAP TRIVIA QUIZ

1. What was Fancy Smith in?...*Z Cars*
2. What was the follow-up show to *Z Cars*?...*Softly, Softly*
3. Which motel was once in a soap?...*Crossroads*
4. Which hospital drama is over 18 years old?...*Casualty*
5. Which two characters have starred in most of the series?...Charlie and Duffy
6. Which soap was based in Liverpool?...*Brookside*
7. Which long-running soap is set in Australia?...*Neighbours*
8. What was the other Australian soap?...*Home and Away*
9. Who starred in *Mother Makes Five*?...Wendy Craig
10. What was the other series she was in?...*Butterflies*
11. Which medical drama is set in the same hospital as *Casualty*?...*Holby City*
12. Which late actor starred in '*Three up, Two down*' and *Eastenders*?...Michael Elphick

13. Which TV station tried to change *News at 10* to 11?...ITV
14. Which Sunday programme is over 25 years old?...*Antiques Roadshow*
15. Which original period drama starred Nyree Dawn Porter?...*Forsyte Saga*
16. Which long-running adaptation of a book had a family whose inherited trait was a grey streak in their hair?...*The Mallens*
17. What was the series set in a boatyard?...*Howard's Way*
18. Who presented *Animal Hospital*?...Rolf Harris
19. What was the prison comedy starring Ronnie Barker?...*Porridge*
20. And the one set in a corner shop?...*Open All Hours*

4. Soap word search

T	H	E	B	I	L	L	Y	O	E
C	O	R	O	N	A	T	I	O	N
S	T	R	E	E	T	D	R	B	M
E	M	M	E	R	D	A	L	E	U
G	I	G	A	W	A	Y	O	R	N
S	R	E	D	N	E	T	S	A	E
C	R	O	S	S	R	O	A	D	S
S	R	E	H	C	R	A	E	H	T
C	A	S	U	A	L	T	Y	T	H
Q	W	F	D	N	A	E	M	O	H

Can you find these words?

THE ARCHERS, HOME AND AWAY, THE BILL, CORONATION STREET, CASUALTY, CROSSROADS, EMMERDALE

5. Each day see how many words can be made from the title of one of the soaps:

- CORONATION STREET
- EASTENDERS
- HOME AND AWAY
- EMMERDALE
- NEIGHBOURS, etc.

Activities for September

Week 1 – Schooldays

Equipment: flipchart, pens, copies of puzzle (or acetate for OHP; see page 174). If staff have old school reports, would they be willing to share them with everyone?

1. Reminiscence and discussion

September is officially the start of the academic year. How old were the clients when they started school? How did they learn to read and write? Did anyone have slate boards? Dip pen and ink, or just pencil? Did they have an ink monitor and what did they do? Did they wear school uniform? Was it hard for the family to afford the uniform? Did they have to wear a certain type of shoes? Did they have school dinners? What were they like? Did they get free milk in the mornings, cod liver oil capsules? Did they have a favourite or hated teacher? Can they remember their name and why they made an impression? Was there bullying at school? Was anyone a victim of bullying? What were the three Rs? (Reading, 'Riting and 'Rithmetic.) Can they remember their tables? Ask for a demonstration. What subjects were they taught? What happened if anyone was left-handed? Was deportment taught? Did they learn anything they are still using today?

Did they get school reports – fortnightly or every term? Did they deliver them unopened to parents? Did they ever forge a signature? What was the worst thing a teacher wrote about them? What was the funniest? Did an adverse comment 'scar' them for life or spur them on to prove it wrong? Does anyone still have their school reports? Did they have a headmaster or mistress? What was their name? Did they have punishments? What were they, and for what misdemeanours were they used? Was anyone in the group punished – if so, for what? What games did they play in the playground? Did they get homework? Did anyone sit the eleven plus? Did anyone win a scholarship? Go to university? Or go to night school to get qualifications? Did they have prefects and head boys/girls? Was anyone a prefect, and what were their duties? Did they go to all boys, girls or mixed schools? What was it like to go up to secondary school from primary school?

Did they have to go to Sunday school? Did they have to help at home when they came back from school? Was there anyone at home when they got in? Can they remember the phrase 'latchkey kids'?

Did anyone win a school prize? For what? Did their school have houses? Can they remember their names and colours?

Does anyone remember the 'nit' nurses visiting? Did anyone get nits, and if so, can they remember the treatment to kill them? Was there a school dentist? Did he put them off dentists for life?

Is anyone still in touch with schoolfriends? Did anyone meet their partner at school? Has anyone heard of Friends Reunited? Who would they like to get in touch with if they could, and why?

Did anyone read comics, e.g. *Beano, Dandy, Eagle, Girl, Bunty, School Friend*? (Make a list and see if the characters' names and descriptions are remembered. Are they still published?) Has anyone still got copies or annuals? Can they bring them in?

How old were they when they left school – and were schooldays the best days of their lives, or is this a myth?

2. Hangman

Use the flipchart and limit words to 'school' items.

3. In my schoolbag I have...

In circle, play the alphabet game.

The first person says, for example, 'In my schoolbag I have an **A**pple.' The next person repeats this and adds an item beginning with B, then the next person adds one with C, and so on, round the group. Encourage the group to assist those who have difficulty, as this improves group cohesion.

4. A schoolboy's desk

Give everyone a copy of the jumbled desk drawer picture (page 174), and if possible use the OHP at the same time. In turn, ask people to verbally pinpoint and identify an object, e.g. 'Bulldog clip, next to the penknife, top lefthand corner.' (Write it on the flipchart to avoid duplication.)

5. See how many words can be made from: PENCIL CASE.

Answers: Pen knife, typing rubber, file tag, key, envelope, pencil sharpener, paper knife, clock, sealing wax, note book, cassette, telephone, filing cabinet, scissors, bulldog clip, ruler, drawing pin, glasses, calendar, wire tray, mug, typewriter, briefcase, ball of string, globe, staples, desk lamp, book, pencil, ink, pen, rubber thimble, paper clip, stamp

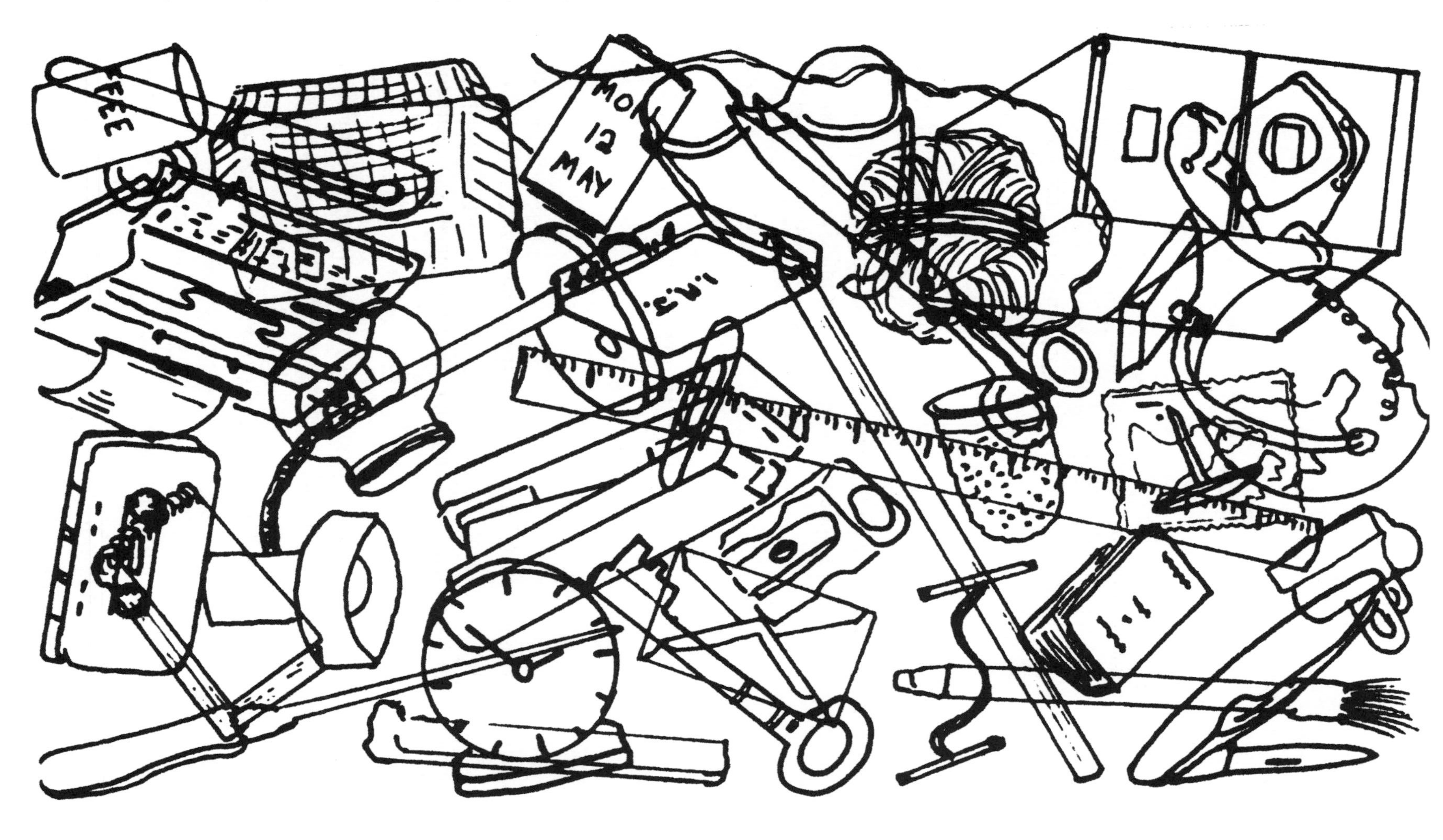

Week 2 – Harvest Festival

Equipment: flipchart, pen, pencils, display of fruits and vegetables – include some exotic ones. Quiz, 'Guess my harvest offering' envelope with names of fruit or veg on pieces of card. Bread, sheaf of corn if possible.

1. Reminiscence and discussion

Can the clients remember past Harvest Festivals? Did they attend Harvest Festivals at church or as part of their school day? Was their school a church school? Where were their local church and school? Can they remember the hymns they sang? Can they still sing them? When they were young, did they live on a farm? Did anyone help to bring the harvest home? Did they get off school to help with this? Did they gather blackberries? Sloes? Did they or their mothers make pickles and preserves? Do they still make jams, marmalade, chutneys and pickles? Any good recipes they can share? When their children were little, can they remember what they sent for the Harvest Festival? Now they are older, are they the recipients of the Harvest Festival offerings from the local church or school?

2. Show the display of fruits and vegetables and ask the group to name them

3. Guess my harvest offering

In two teams, taking turns to guess. A team member selects a card from the envelope and shows it to his or her team. The opposing team has three questions to guess what is on the card (name of a fruit or vegetable). The questions can be answered by the first team only with a 'yes' or 'no'. If the guessing team guesses correctly, they win three points. If not, the points are awarded to the opposing team. Try to ensure that each team member has a turn selecting a card.

4. A Green Grocery List

Still in teams, write down as many fruits and veg as they can think of in ten minutes. The winning team could be awarded a grape each!

5. CHOPPED VEGETABLES

Write the anagrams on the flipchart.

PSOETTAO	potatoes	PSAE	peas
CTAORR	carrot	GUSARPSNA-SAPE	sugarsnap peas
SEWED	swede	RECAWUOLLIF	cauliflower
PIRNASP	parsnip	IBLROOCC	broccoli
NNIOO	onion	ECTOTUERG	courgette
SWETENCOR	sweetcorn	DBARO SBNEA	broad beans
BTEOTOER	beetroot	RREUNN SBNEA	runner beans
SSPROTU	sprouts	CGIALR	garlic
BSNEA	beans		

6. Vegetable guess

(from *More Mental Aerobics* page 273)

What vegetables do we eat the:

- stems of?...asparagus, celery, leeks
- seeds of?...peas, beans, corn
- leaves of?...lettuce, cabbage, spinach, watercress, sprouts
- flowers of?...broccoli, cauliflower
- fruit of?...tomato, pepper, courgette, aubergine
- root of?...radish, beetroot, carrot, onion, parsnip, turnip

7. Harvest feely bag

Put different vegetables and fruits in a bag. Pass the bag to each client in turn and ask them to feel inside it and identify what they are feeling, by writing it down if possible. When all have had a turn, score the answers by showing the contents of the bag.

8. See how many words can be made from: HARVEST HOME.

Week 3 – What's in a name?

Equipment: flipchart, pens, example of names from the Births announcements page of the local paper, book on the meanings of names, copies of 'Famous people in a muddle' (page 180) and picture quizzes (page 182).

1. Reminiscence and discussion

Ask everyone their full names, *including* their middle names. Why were they called that? Is it a family name? Were they named after someone? A family member or someone famous? Does anyone have a name they dislike? What would they have preferred to be called? Do they think their name suits them? Do they like their surname? What was their maiden name? Has anyone changed their name by deed poll? Does anyone know people who have an apt name for their profession/job, e.g. Mr Stone the builder? Can they think of any famous people with the same name as themselves? Does anyone have a nickname? Did they have one when they were young?

On the flipchart write everyone's names to see which are the most popular. Does anyone know what their name means? Tell everyone the meaning of their name. Does it match their personality? Or did they grow to match their name?

Names change in popularity over time. Can they think of old-fashioned names that are enjoying a new lease of life? What do they think about the names famous people give their children, e.g. Trixie-Bell, Brooklyn, Tuesday, Moonwalker (add more)? What about the people who name their children after soap stars – are they sorry for children with 'daft' names? Is life made unnecessarily hard for them? Brooklyn Beckham was named after the place he was conceived. If they had to be named after the places they were conceived or born, what would they be called? Can they think of some funny names people could have if they were conceived in odd sounding places? Accrington Stanley, Middle Wallop, Fizackerly, etc.

2. Name that famous person

(based on *Mental Aerobics* page 29)

Either give the famous person's name and ask what they were famous for, or give the description and ask for their name. Play in teams, or as a general quiz.

1. Emperor of France...Napoleon
2. Wrote *The Origin of Species*...Charles Darwin
3. Silent actor, played a tramp...Charlie Chaplin
4. Fashion designer, famous perfume No.5...Chanel (Coco)
5. Naval hero, badly injured, kissed Hardy...Horatio Nelson
6. Famous British Prime Minister of World War II...Churchill
7. Film star famous for her legs...Betty Grable

8. Wrote many novels that had a social impact, e.g. *Oliver Twist*...Charles Dickens
9. A king gave up his throne for her, famous divorcée...Wallis Simpson
10. Member of the Rat Pack, nick named Ol' Blue Eyes, singer...Frank Sinatra
11. Burned at the stake, girl warrior...Joan of Arc
12. A fiddler in the flames, cruel ruler of Rome...Nero
13. Married a King who had her beheaded, mother of the most famous Queen...Anne Boleyn
14. Egyptian pharaoh, his golden body covering has been seen by millions...Tutankamen
15. Most photographed face, tragic figure, died in a car crash in France...Princess Diana
16. Played a chandelier-bedecked piano, wore fantastic outfits and loved his mother...Liberace
17. His 'swingometer' was just a bit of fun and a feature of many elections...Peter Snow
18. Yorkshire bowler who was fiery...Fred Truman
19. Poet of the Lake District who liked daffodils...William Wordsworth
20. Crusader King, bravehearted, had a brother called John...Richard the Lionheart
21. Disney character with big black ears, loves Minnie and has a club...Mickey Mouse

3. Famed for...

Who was associated with the following?

1. The *Santa Maria*...Columbus
2. A cigar...Churchill
3. A trumpet and a hanky...Louis Armstrong
4. An apple and a snake...Eve
5. A flood...Noah
6. A long sleep...Rip van Winkle
7. A glass slipper...Cinderella
8. A burning bush...Moses
9. A spider's web...Robert the Bruce
10. A coat of many colours...Joseph

Add more of your own.

4. Names anagrams

Give everyone a paper and pencil for individual work. Write the anagrams on the flipchart. Staff/clients' names can be added to the list.

SEOR	Rose	ASONLI	Alison
YNANHOT	Anthony	MELLICHE	Michelle
YDOORTH	Dorothy	DAINL	Linda
NDEERO	Doreen	AADMAN	Amanda
RALAU	Laura	CEHNRIST	Christine
YELIM	Emily	JEUIL	Julie
HDALOR	Harold	LYNARCO	Carolyn
SHELCAR	Charles	NIBRA	Brian
FALDER	Alfred	MEJSA	James
RHYEN	Henry	RIEC	Eric
IDDAV	David	THNEKNE	Kenneth
CHILAME	Michael	PESHTCRORIH	Christopher

5. Who's who?

Can you name the six people in the bus queue, given the following clues? * Oliver is looking for the bus. * Jack and Leo are the tallest and shortest. * If Rosie was on the right of Rachel they would be back to back. * Amy is talking to Jack.

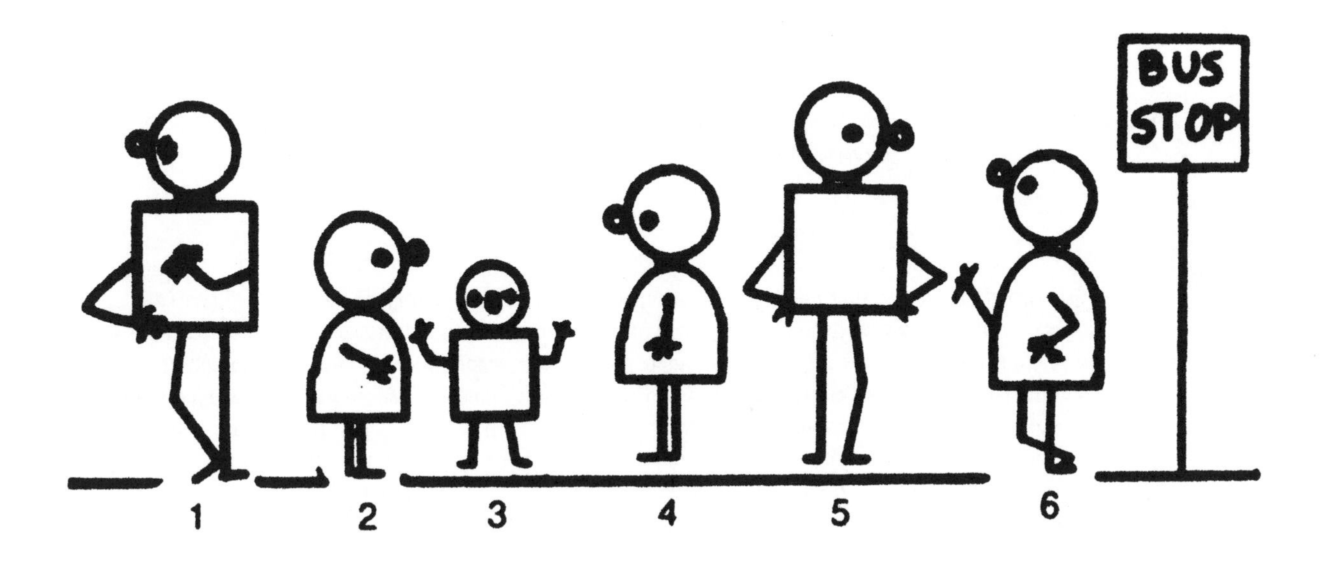

Answers: 1 .Oliver 2 .Rosie 3 . Leo 4. Rachel 5. Jack 6. Amy

6. Famous people in a muddle

Fit the correct descriptions (one from each coloumn) to these famous people.

Queen Victoria	lived at 10 Downing Street	was the founder of modern nursing	lives in Buckingham Palace
Winston Churchill	his woman was Eve	his sons were Ham, Shem and Japheth	is the Bishop of Rome
Adolf Hitler	built an Ark	was the first man in the Bible	lived at Chartwell
Florence Nightingale	was married to Prince Albert	lives at the Vatican	acted in *National Velvet*
Adam	is the head of the Catholic Church	sat in the House of Commons	was the first British woman Prime Minister
Noah	led Germany in the 2nd World War	was an accomplished painter	lived in the Garden of Eden
Queen Elizabeth II	was sister to the Queen	a London railway station bears her name	had a small moustache
The Pope	led Britain in World War II	is a famous film star	took in 2 animals of each species
Princess Margaret	is married to the Duke of Edinburgh	is mother of the heir to the throne	her surname is that of a songbird
Elizabeth Taylor	was a nurse in the Crimean War	her second name is Rose	is the great grandmother of Elizabeth II
Margaret Thatcher	has been married several times – twice to the same man	committed suicide in a bunker	her son is Viscount Linley

Answers: Queen Victoria...was married to Prince Albert...a London railway station bears her name...is the great grandmother of Elizabeth II; Winston Churchill...led Britain in World War II...was an accomplished painter...lived at Chartwell; Adolf Hitler...led Germany in World War II...committed suicide in a bunker...had a small moustache; Florence Nightingale...was a nurse in the Crimean War...was the founder of modern nursing...her surname is that of a songbird; Adam...his woman was Eve...was the first man in the Bible...lived in the Garden of Eden; Noah...built an Ark...his sons were Ham, Shem and Japheth...took in 2 animals of each species; Queen Elizabeth II...is married to the Duke of Edinburgh...is mother of the heir to the throne...lives in Buckingham Palace; The Pope...is the head of the Catholic Church...lives at the Vatican...is the Bishop of Rome; Princess Margaret...was sister to the Queen...her second name is Rose...her son is Viscount Linley; Elizabeth Taylor...has been married several times – twice to the same man...is a famous film star...acted in *National Velvet*; Margaret Thatcher...lived at 10 Downing Street...sat in the House of Commons...was the first British woman Prime Minister

7. Male/female and their young

Ask the group in general

a male cow...*bull*

a male hen...*cock*

a young sheep...*lamb*

a young horse...*foal*

a young cat...*kitten*

a young dog...*puppy*

a female lion...*lioness*

a young goat...*kid*

a female dog...*bitch*

a young tiger...*cub*

a female goat...*nanny*

female equivalent of Cub scout...*Brownie*

female equivalent of a duke...*duchess*

female equivalent of a bachelor...*spinster*

a female actor...*actress*

a female fox...*vixen*

a female sheep...*ewe*

a male horse...*stallion*

a female peacock...*peahen*

a young deer...*fawn*

a young goose...*gosling*

a male witch...*wizard*

a male rabbit...*buck*

a male pig...*boar*

a young elephant...*calf*

a young frog...*tadpole*

a young eel...*elver*

female equivalent of nephew...*niece*

And a few harder ones:

a female ferret...*gill*

a female marquis...*marchioness*

a young hare...*leveret*

a young seal...*pup*

a young wasp...*grub*

a female badger...*sow*

a young trout...*fry*

a male swan...*cob*

a female sultan...*sultana*

a male equivalent of heifer...*steer*

8. Relatively speaking

What relation is Pat to Jane

That girl Pat is my niece.
Yes, but she is not my niece.
Is Dick married?
No he is Jane's brother.
DICK
JANE
JOHN
PAT

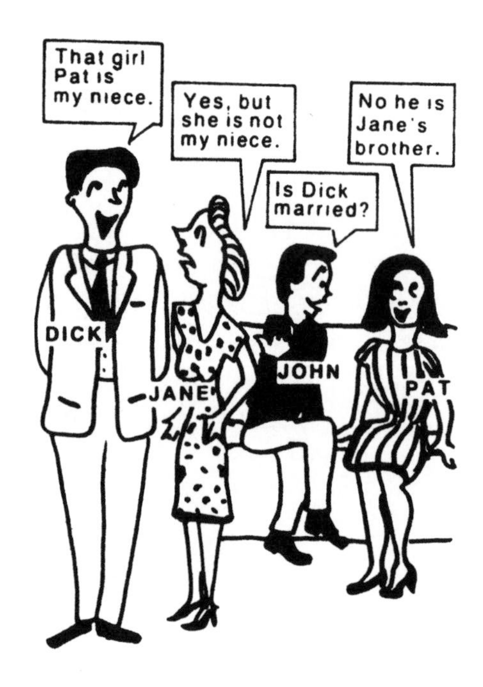

Answer: Pat is Jane's daughter.

9. See how many words can be made from: DAVID BECKHAM

(or the name of a member of staff).

Week 4 – Autumn

Equipment: collect different fallen leaves, nuts, fruits, seeds, fungi, ears of corn, conkers, paint colour charts, autumnal pictures, autumn poems, Kim's Game trays, giant pumpkin.

1. Reminiscence and discussion

Ask what autumn means to the group? Walks in the woods? Falling leaves – are they seen as a thing of beauty or a nuisance (extra work to clear them, train delays, even dangerous when slippery and wet)? When young, did they help with ploughing? Apple picking? Mushrooming, collecting firewood, conkers? Sweeping leaves, burning dead wood, etc.? Does anyone know what the Americans call autumn? Why do they call it 'fall'? (Leaf fall.) Has anyone been to Canada in the fall?

Did or do they make preserves to see them through the winter? Jams – what kind? Pickles – what did they use? Chutney? What other ways of preserving food can they think of? (Salting, smoking, drying, freezing, canning.) Can anyone remember anything else that would be done to prepare for winter? (Fuel stores, log piles.) Did they change their summer curtains for winter-quality ones?

Read some autumn poems, especially Keats' 'Ode to Autumn'. You may also find some in magazines.

Show the leaf collection – can anyone recognise the different leaves? (Don't forget to label them!) Guess the weight of the giant pumpkin and ask if anyone has made pumpkin pie, or tasted it. Perhaps one could be made to try.

2. Autumn grammar game

(based on *More Mental Aerobics* page 263)

People are familiar with nouns – words to denote a person, place or thing – but maybe not so with adjectives – words that are used to describe a noun. Either individually or in teams, give an autumnal noun and ask for an adjective from the clients.

NOUNS	ADJECTIVES
sunset	orange, crimson
corn	ripened, plump, yellow, golden
nuts	brown, shiny, polished, knobbly, hard
grapes	purple, green, plump, sweet, juicy
bonfire	warm, glowing, roaring, crackling, sparking, smoky
fragrance	wood-scented, mouldy
crops	full-grown, bounteous, harvested
mist	damp, hazy
winds	chill, howling, blustery
smoke	blue-hazed, wood-scented
hills	smoky, hazy, frosty, distant
clouds	fleecy, drifting, dark, laden
air	clean, crisp, scented, pure
scarecrow	lonely, bedraggled, funny
fields	muddy, stubbled, ploughed, dying back
leaves	golden, brown, red, swirling, rustling, dry, crunching
frost	hoar, white, cold, crackly
squirrels	scurrying, busy, forgetful
sheaves	golden, corny
seeds	sweet, life-bearing, golden, ripe

earth	resting, rich, brown, waiting
rain	heavy, sudden, pelting
moon	harvest, white, pale yellow
trees	leafless, bare, branched
apples	red, green, juicy, polished
days	shortening, brisk, chilly, crisp

3. Autumn 'what am I?'

(based on *More Mental Aerobics* page 265)

Ask the group in turn. Assistance may be given by the rest of the group.

Three or four clues are given for each item. Give the first clue and allow time for an answer, if incorrect give the second clue, and so on. Add more clues of your own or ask the clients to add some.

1. My insides are soft and seedy.
   I make a scary face.
   Peter liked to eat me.
   pumpkin

2. I flower in autumn.
   My name is difficult to spell.
   I have many petals.
   I come in many colours.
   chrysanthemum

3. I like nuts.
   I hide my winter stores.
   I have a curved, fluffy tail.
   I am a nimble tree climber.
   squirrel

4. I make a crunchy carpet.
   I have wonderful autumn colours.
   Deciduous trees lose me.
   leaves

5. I am shiny and brown.
   I am prized by boys.
   There is a 'horse' and a sweet variety of me.
   chestnuts

12. My bundles are stood in rows.
    I am used to store dried food.
    I am often stored in a barn.
    'Giant' was a wrestler.
    haystacks

13. I am fragile.
    I look like lace.
    I catch the frost and raindrops.
    My maker has eight legs.
    spider's web

14. I am made from apples.
    I come in a bottle.
    Some call me scrumpy.
    cider

15. I happen in October.
    I have become Americanised.
    A game of mine is bobbing for apples.
    halloween

16. I come more often at this time.
    I cover leaves and webs.
    I make water hard.
    frost

6. I am full of sweet juice.
   People stomp on me.
   I often accompany a meal.
   I grow on a vine.
   grapes

7. I swim.
   I fly in a 'V' formation, sometimes a skein.
   I honk.
   goose

8. I have a scent.
   I drift in a grey-blue haze.
   I come from a fire.
   smoke

9. When I am popped, you can buy me at the cinema.
   I make bread.
   I have ears.
   corn

10. I am a sphere.
    I can be red, green or golden.
    I can be pressed for a drink.
    apple

11. I am very tall.
    I face the sun.
    I have edible seeds.
    I can make oil.
    I have bright yellow petals.
    sunflower

17. My anniversary comes in late autumn.
    I am associated with the Houses of Parliament.
    I go with a bang.
    I have a code of safety.
    Guy Fawkes Night/Bonfire Night

18. I grow in hedgerows.
    I can scratch.
    I make a wonderful pie.
    blackberry

19. I till the fields ready for planting.
    In the Bible swords were made into me.
    I save farmers lots of time.
    plough

20. I shine white.
    Men have walked on me.
    I wax and wane.
    Lovers love me.
    moon

21. I attract the birds.
    I am often made of wood.
    Nuts, bread and fat can be found on me.
    I am found in the garden.
    bird table

4. Sensory autumn

(from *More Mental Aerobics* page 271)

On the flipchart write the headings **Sight** – **Sound** – **Smell** – **Touch** – **Taste**. Ask the group to suggest autumnal words for each category, and list them.

Sight: gold, russet, rust, red, orange, yellow, crimson, brown, tan, magenta, hazy, flickering, sparking, whirling, glowing, dark, etc.

Sound: crackle, crunch, rustle, blustery, chopping, howling, gusty, laughter (of children kicking leaves), etc.

Smell: mouldy, mushroom, acrid, smoky, spicy, scented, fermenting, dank, etc.

Touch: dry, crisp, chilly, wet, nippy, damp, slippery, etc.

Taste: sweet, sour, vinegary, sugary, spicy, tart, salty, bitter, etc.

Have samples of items that fit into the categories, such as cinnamon sticks, mushrooms, hazelnuts, blackberries, crisp red apples, dry leaves... Invite people to handle them and involve their senses in the activity.

5. Autumn colours

Encourage the group to list the colours of autumn. Paint shops will give you colour charts to assist. Enjoy the inventive names given by the manufacturers to colours like rust, russet, gold, wine, chestnut, tan...

6. Autumn brainstorm poem

On the flipchart pin a large, autumnal scene and entitle it 'How we see autumn'.

Go round the group and ask each person for a word or phrase that springs to mind when they look at the picture of autumn. Write the words in a column under the picture, ending with '...is our autumn.' Then read it out as a group poem, if it flows well. Otherwise, just continue to add to the list. *Example*: 'frosty, leaves, rustling, crunchy, shadowy, musty, toadstool, ripening, apples, nuts hidden, school days starting, children playing, is our autumn.'

If the group wishes, ask them to write their own poem. Here is an example of one written by Queens Court group:

Autumn Thursday

Red berries on the trees
Confusing all the wasps and bees
White clouds and skies of blue
Summer's over Autumn's due.

Brown leaves on the floor
Autumn's knocking on the door
The rustic charm of Autumn days
Peep at you through frosty haze.

Fallen fruit to pick and store
Behind the bulging pantry door
Golden apples fresh and sweet

Good enough for all to eat.

Blackberries, elderberries, cranberries too
Baked in a pie for me and you
Frosty mornings, Autumn's mist
All are part of Autumn's list.

The Queens Court Thursday Group

7. Autumn Kim's Game

In two groups, one tray per group.

Put a number of fruits, nuts and leaves on each tray. Allow the clients two minutes to look at the tray, remove it from sight and ask them to recall what is on the tray. Bring it back to check results, then remove from sight once more and take one item away. Bring it back again to the clients and see how many tell correctly what is missing. List responses, then ask how they remembered the item – shape? Size? Colour? Position on tray?

Week 5 – Newspapers and current affairs

Equipment: flipchart, pens, newspapers including local paper, laminated pictures of 'celebrities', copies of 'Newspaper' word search (page 189), newspaper cartoon books.

1. Reminiscence and discussion

Ask if clients get a newspaper every day, just at weekends, or never. Where do they get their news from? TV, radio, newspapers? Which paper do they read? Have they always read the same paper? Why do they prefer that paper? Is it the one their parents/spouse introduced them to? Can people name the newspapers on sale today? Can they name the ones no longer in print? (List titles on the flipchart.)

Can people recognise the particular political slants of the newspapers? What do they think of the *Sun*, *Mirror*, *Star*, *News of the World* and the *Sunday Sport*? Does anyone read a broadsheet? Do they think *The Times* has been reduced in standing, as well as size? What do they think of all the wasted paper in the endless supplements and inserts? Do they ever read them? Do they have a paper delivered? Do they feel sorry for the paper delivery boys and girls having to carry such a lot of heavy paper in their bags? Did any of them ever have a paper round?

Do they think the newspapers tell us the truth? Do journalists sensationalise everything in a cynical way to sell papers? Are the papers just filled with doom and gloom, or is life really like that today? Do they feel that newspapers have had to change how they present their news because we now have 24-hour news on TV? Do the media have to sensationalise everything and give us more details than we require? Does the group feel the journalists are too intrusive? Who do they believe – the newspapers or TV?

Do they still read the local newspaper? Do they always read the births, deaths and marriages? Have they used it to sell anything? Read the 'Lonely Hearts' column? Have they ever appeared in a newspaper? How did the printed story differ from what they had said to the reporter? Has this made them less likely to believe what they read? Do people prefer to read a magazine rather than a newspaper? List the magazines they used to read, and the current ones.

Does everyone like to read their horoscope? Is it ever true?

Do people read the cartoons in the papers? Do they think this is a good way of getting your message across? Show some such as Giles, Matt, etc., from the cartoon annuals. Can they remember the ones when they were young, such as Andy Capp, and the ones especially for youngsters, like Rupert Bear and Flook?

Do people like to do the crossword puzzles and quizzes? Can anyone do Sudoku? Ask everyone if they can remember what have been the main news stories in the past week. What do they think about the way ordinary people are destroyed by the media when their story is splashed all over the papers, then forgotten the next week, and they are left with their lives in pieces? Is it a British trait that they build people up just to knock them down? (Name some fallen idols.) Do they feel sorry for the 'celebrities' who are 'doorstepped' and hounded by the news photographers?

2. Listen carefully

Look at the headlines in a current paper, then select a story – either an interesting feature or a news article. Tell the clients to listen carefully, as you will ask ten questions relating to the article. Read the article loudly and clearly, then ask the relevant questions.

TRY THE DAILY CROSSWORD

Copy a newspaper's crossword onto the flipchart and read out the clues for group completion.

3. Recycling

Ask the clients what old newspapers were (and still can be) used for. Some prompts: toilet paper, dog training, relining shoes, recycling newsprint paper, *firelighters*. Give everyone a sheet of newspaper and ask them to fold a firelighter like the ones they made in their youth. (Some folk may also make a spell, which is a thin roll of paper, used like a match, to light things from a fire.) It is interesting to see how people from different parts of the country make firelighters particular to their area. Try the following newspaper activities:

- Torn paper-doll chains – some people may still remember how to fold and make these.
- Make a hat from a folded newspaper.

Any other ideas people have for newspapers?

4. Celebrities quiz

Pass the pictures of celebrities around the group. Ask who they are and the reason for their being a celebrity – do they really deserve to be famous?

5. Newspaper word search

D	A	I	L	Y	P	A	P	E	R	S	E
P	A	E	L	C	I	N	O	R	H	C	X
M	I	R	R	O	R	V	D	A	B	S	P
J	T	N	L	O	I	L	P	U	U	P	R
M	U	T	I	M	E	S	R	C	X	O	E
S	T	A	D	T	Y	M	O	W	T	R	S
T	E	L	E	G	R	A	P	H	O	T	S
A	F	H	U	P	J	I	Y	O	N	R	D
R	I	N	F	V	H	L	O	I	D	N	P
G	U	A	R	D	I	A	N	E	W	S	U
E	V	E	N	I	N	G	M	K	A	P	Z
I	N	D	E	P	E	N	D	E	N	T	L

Can you find these in the grid?

DAILY PAPERS, EXPRESS, TELEGRAPH, MIRROR, STAR, INDEPENDENT, SUN, MAIL, GUARDIAN, SPORT, TIMES, CHRONICLE, EVENING NEWS

6. See how many words can be made from: READ ALL ABOUT IT!

Activities for October

Week 1 – Healthy body, healthy mind

See if you can get a nurse, pharmacist, health visitor, occupational therapist or physiotherapist to give a talk on their particular profession and about maintaining good health and avoiding falls as we get older.

Equipment: flipchart, pens, body quiz, two pairs of clear glasses – one pair smeared with Vaseline, one pair with both lenses half-covered on the left side with paper, relaxation tape, relaxing music.

1. Reminiscence and discussion

With winter coming on, talk about how to remain healthy, the importance of good diet, keeping warm, flu jabs (ask who will have one – maybe a chance to arrange this). Maybe a community nurse or local pharmacist would come and give a talk on health and the importance of medication. Does anyone have their medication delivered? Is it in a prepacked medi-dose box? Do people ask the pharmacist if they are buying over-the-counter medication and are on prescribed medication? (They should.) Do they think that if they can buy medication over the counter, it is not as strong as what the doctor prescribes and won't react with their prescribed medicine? Does anyone use herbal remedies? Which? Do they think we use too many antibiotics? Is this wise, in view of the superbugs?

What sort of remedies did their parents use? Did they have to comply with old wives' tales when they were young? Which? (For example, not washing their hair when menstruating, 'feed a cold and starve a fever', don't pick dandelions (they make you wee), 'having a road through you' once a week (sulphur and molasses to make their bowels open. Some people have had their natural bowel movements completely disrupted by this practice and now require almost daily anti-constipation medication).) Do they know any of the old remedies that are back in fashion? (Maggots are being used for ulcers, leeches are being used again, honey on wounds.)

How did their mother treat earache, toothache, headache, colds and flu, stomach upsets? Did they have any serious childhood illnesses? How were they treated?

Can anyone remember when the National Health Service began? How did they see a doctor before, how did they pay? Was there a local wise woman who helped with ill health and childbirth? Did anyone pay weekly at work for health care? Does anyone use private health care? Is it better, or just quicker then the NHS? Has anyone been in hospital? What was it like? Has it changed from when they were young? What were the doctors and nurses like? Were they over worked? Do they think the old-fashioned Matron was a good idea? Do they have any funny stories about hospital? Do they think you get better more quickly at home? Has anyone had to go to casualty? Taken their children? Where did they have their children – at home or in hospital?

Do they think men are not very good at looking after themselves? Are reluctant to go to a doctor? Make poor patients? Does everyone feel reluctant to call out the doctor? When was the last time they did this? How was it received by the surgery? Can everyone give their best tip for staying healthy?

The words 'health' and 'wholeness' come from the same Old Saxon and Early English roots, words like *hail, hool, heil* (like 'hale and hearty') which mean 'unwounded, entire, sound', showing that we have ancient concepts of health encompassing both mind and body, so that disease (dis-ease) in one has a knock-on effect in the other.

2. 'Know your body' quiz

(based on *More Mental Aerobics* page 46)

1. Marrow is found in which part of the body?...bone
2. What part of the digestive system leads from the throat to the stomach?...oesophagus
3. These organs remove urea from the body...kidneys
4. Name the five senses...sight, smell, hearing, taste and touch
5. Which organ pumps your blood?...heart
6. What is another term for procreate?...reproduce
7. Which is the largest organ?...skin
8. Which organ is found in the skull?...brain
9. Where two bones come together, it is a...joint
10. Which blood cells carry oxygen?...red
11. This word means the transfer of characteristics from our parents...heredity
12. Its loss can be a source of anxiety to men!...hair
13. These contract to give us mobility...muscles
14. This system coordinates all the body's activities in response to signals...nervous system
15. This is the framework of the body...skeleton
16. This nerve pain runs down the back of the leg...sciatica

17. These organs hold air...lungs
18. This organ secretes bile ...liver
19. The tailbone in the spine is the...coccyx
20. What process converts food for nourishment and energy?...digestion
21. This cord runs inside the vertebrae...spinal
22. Which blood cells help the immune system?...white
23. What can be rhesus positive?...blood
24. The body has how many pints of blood – 5, 10 or 25?...10
25. Chewed food is lubricated by what?...saliva
26. What can be caused by too much gastric acid?...ulcer
27. This organ is soft, grey, and looks like a cauliflower...brain
28. For what do we use the cochlea, Eustachian tube and tympani?...hearing
29. What has over 1300 nerve endings per square inch?...fingertip
30. What are the four primary tastes we experience?...sweet, sour, salty, bitter
31. The human gestation period is...9 months
32. What is the normal body temperature?...98.6°F (37°C)
33. What is the body mostly made up of?...water
34. The largest artery is...aorta
35. Which part of the face is used mainly in smelling?...nose
36. Insulin-producing cells are in this gland...pancreas
37. A deficiency of iron causes what?...anaemia
38. Molars, canine, incisors and wisdom are...teeth
39. What substance clogs the arteries?...cholesterol
40. All living matter consists of these basic building blocks...cells
41. What was used to cure most illnesses in the olden days?...bloodletting
42. What at the end of the colon is removed when enflamed?...appendix
43. Where we get digitalis, used for treating the heart...foxglove
44. The body, less limbs and head, is known as the...torso, trunk
45. Can you identify adam's apple, bellybutton, funnybone, earlobe, nape of the neck, gullet, patella (kneecap), pinky, crook of the arm, solar plexus?

3. 'With a song in my heart'

On the flipchart list any songs with body parts in them – and sing them!

Some starters (based on *More Mental Aerobics* page 48):

- Heart of my Heart.
- My Heart belongs to Daddy.
- When Irish Eyes are Smiling.
- Five Feet Two, Eyes of Blue.

- Dear Hearts and Gentle People.
- Angel Eyes.
- I left my Heart in San Francisco.
- Jeannie with the Light Brown Hair.
- I'm Gonna Wash that Man Right out of my Hair.
- Ma, he's making Eyes at me.
- Smoke gets in your Eyes.
- I've got You under my Skin.
- Put your Head on my Shoulder.
- He's got the Whole World in His Hands.
- Your Tiny Hand is Frozen.
- Georgia on my Mind.
- Baby Face.
- Put on a Happy Face.

4. Exercise for a healthy body

Does anyone remember the Green Goddess? Rosemary Conley? To get the blood flowing play the following action songs – use a different one each day.

- The Hokey Cokey. This can be done sitting down – apart from 'turn around'! So say, 'Turn your head from side to side' and for 'Kiss me in the middle' say, 'Oh, stamp your feet and clap your hands.'
- Heads, Shoulders, Knees and Toes.
- Dem Bones, dem Bones.
- Simon says...

5. Empathy

Discuss how some people have to cope with being disabled by illness, and ask if anyone would like to experience what they have to cope with, and how.

- Ask people to try to write their names with their non-dominant hand, and then to draw a house, a flower and a clockface. This simulates the effects of a stroke.
- Smear some clear glasses with Vaseline. This is what it's like to have a cataract.
- Half-cover some clear glasses with paper on the left side of both lenses. This is how a person sees the world with 'neglect' following a stroke.
- If you have some fluid thickener, make some up in tea and see who is willing to try a sip...not many! This is how people who lose their swallow reflex after a stroke have to drink.

6. Bodily expressions

(based on *More Mental Aerobics* page 110)

Ask the group to fill in the part of the body in the expressions. Read them out, missing out the words in square brackets.

1. You have a good [head] on your shoulders.
2. Use a little [elbow] grease.
3. Put your [shoulder] to the wheel.
4. Swivel [hips].
5. Honey [lips].
6. He's a pain in the [neck].
7. If you twist my [arm]...
8. You're pulling my [leg].
9. The two go [hand]-in-[hand].
10. He's under the [thumb] of...
11. Is he bending your [ear]?
12. Best [foot] forward.
13. You are the apple of my [eye].
14. [Foot] loose and fancy free.
15. Motor [mouth].
16. The [hand] is quicker than the [eye].
17. Have a [heart].
18. [Heart]-to-[heart].
19. Get your [teeth] into it.
20. Shake a [leg].
21. Grease my [palm].
22. Lose [face].
23. [Heart] in my mouth.
24. Keep [body] and soul together.
25. Pay [lip] service.
26. One [foot] in the grave.

7. 'Show a leg' quiz

Ask members of the group in turn to mime or gesture the answers to this quiz.

1. A giraffe has a long one...neck
2. Away of showing pleasure when at the theatre...clap hands
3. –, – and boomps-a-daisy...hands, knees
4. What does a comb have?...teeth
5. Twelve inches make?...a foot
6. A stem of corn is called an...ear
7. A Member of Parliament has one...seat
8. What is hit by a hammer?...nail
9. Children like to eat fish ones...fingers
10. Onions make you...cry
11. In war, men are called to...arms
12. In Bingo it's – eleven...legs
13. Dates grown on this...palm
14. Where was Achilles vulnerable?...heel
15. A cheeky person gives a lot of...lip
16. To shun someone you give a cold...shoulder
17. This makes things stick...gum

18. When you toss for it, you call '– or tails'...heads
19. Underneath the spreading – tree...chestnut
20. Put your – to the grindstone...shoulder
21. The way to signal 'yes' and 'no'...nod and shake head
22. When you want obedience you say '– the line'...toe
23. – up, Mother Brown...knees

8. A healthy mind

Stress is one of the main causes of tiredness and ill health, so it is important to learn to relax and reduce stress levels. Make sure everyone is sitting in a comfortable position with their feet on the floor, back supported, hands on knees, and can hear you. Ask them to close their eyes. Then *either* play a relaxation tape *or*:

Ask everyone to breathe slowly and deeply, getting into a nice, even rhythm, slowing right down, breathing in through their nose and out through their mouth. Do this for a few minutes and then ask them to envisage their favourite flower, see it very clearly: all the petals, the leaves, even see a drop of dew on the petals and maybe a ladybird, a butterfly or bee sitting in the centre. (This is to fill the mind and help people to switch off from their worries.) After about seven or eight minutes of relaxation, ask them to gently move their fingers and toes, then, still breathing slowly and deeply, gently open their eyes and slowly come back to the here and now. Remind them to get up slowly when they come to stand, as their blood pressure will have dropped and they may get dizzy.

Ask if everyone is relaxed and if they enjoyed the sensation. If yes, tell them it is a good way of getting off to sleep at night. If they really enjoyed it they may want to do it more often in the group.

9. Why worry?

There are only two things to worry about; either you are well or you are sick.
If you are well, there is nothing to worry about.
But if you are sick, there are only two things to worry about.
Either you will get well; or you will die.
If you get well, there is nothing to worry about.
But if you die, there are only two things to worry about.
Either you will go to Heaven or you will go to Hell.
If you go to Heaven, there is nothing to worry about.
But if you go to Hell –
You'll be so busy shaking hands with friends that you won't have time to worry.

10. See how many words can be made from: NATIONAL HEALTH SERVICE.

Week 2 – Animals and pets

Equipment: flipchart, pens. Perhaps some pets could be brought in.

1. Reminiscence and discussion

Ask the group if they had pets when they were young. What were they, and what were their names? If they were not allowed a pet, which animal would they have loved to have? Do they have any stories – funny, sad or heroic – that they could share about their pets? Do they have a pet now? What? Does any member of their family have pets? What? Does anyone they know have an exotic animal? What pets do children today have? Did anyone have a tortoise? A goldfish from the fair or from the rag-and-bone man?

Does the group enjoy the animal programmes on TV? Who is their favourite presenter? Can they remember Johnny Morris and George Cansdale, the first presenters on children's television? Armand and Michaela Denis? Jacques Cousteau? Are they impressed with the fantastic camerawork in today's animal programmes? Which wild animal do they like the best? Make a list. Are they all the furry, cuddly ones? Why? Which wild animals did they like when they were young? Anyone like insects? Creepy crawlies? Frogs?

Did they go to the zoo when they were young? Have they been lately? Has it changed? How? Zoos now do more to help endangered species. What is the World Wildlife Fund (WWF)'s logo? (Panda.) Is anyone a member of the WWF? Is anyone in the RSPCA? Do they give to animal protection societies? What do they think of people who leave bequests to cats' and dogs' homes? What is the famous dog rescue home in London? (Battersea.)

Has anyone been to the circus? Has that changed since they were young? Is this so much better? How do people feel about animals used in magic tricks, and the monkeys used by foreign street photographers? Donkeys at the seaside? Bull- and cock-fighting, fox-hunting, big game hunters, ivory poachers, Chinese medicine which asks for tiger bone and the bile of bears (who are kept in captivity so this can be tapped)? Factory farming? Battery-farmed hens?

Animals have been used to enhance our lives for thousands of years. Can people list the ways? Herding sheep/cattle, guarding, police dogs (sniffer dogs for drugs and explosives), search-and-rescue dogs (in the war they were used to locate fallen soldiers and people in bombed houses), message-carrying dogs and pigeons, Guide Dogs for the Blind, hearing dogs, dogs who sense when epileptic fits are about to happen, pat dogs in some residential settings for reducing stress. And for *companionship*...complete, unconditional love.

People usually divide into cat or dog lovers. See if this is the case with the group, and ask to hear the reasons for their preferences. Tell the following homily and see if they agree:

> A dog was kept by a man who fed him, cared for him and gave him shelter.
> 'The Man is a God,' thought the dog.
>
> A cat was kept by a man who fed him, cared for him and gave him shelter.
> '*I* am a God,' thought the cat!

2. Mammal Quiz

(based on *More Mental Aerobics* page 57)

Definition: A mammal is warm-blooded, has hair, and the females feed their young with milk. Ask the group in general:

1. I live in all the oceans of the world.
I feed on fish and squid.
I can leap into the air and somersault.
I navigate by echo-location.
I am related to the porpoise.
dolphin

2. I am a member of the weasel family.
I love salt and fresh water and can live on land.
I made a 'Ring of Bright Water'.
I love salmon but will eat all fish, frogs and sea animals.
I have luxurious fur.
otter

3. I can be black, brown or grey.
I am universally disliked.
I am a rodent.
It is said you are never more than a few feet away from one of us.
A Pied Piper was once used instead of Warfarin to exterminate us.
The Black Plague is linked with me.
rat

4. I am the largest member of the deer family.
I have very large antlers.
I live in Canada.
moose

5. I live only in Australia.
My muzzle is shaped like a duck's beak.
My tail is like a beaver's.
platypus

16. Davy Crockett made a hat from me!
I have a ringed tail and a mask.
I live in America.
raccoon

17. I have a hump.
The North American Indians hunted me.
I have horns.
I am a member of the cattle family.
bison/buffalo

18. I have large tusks.
The biggest male is known as the beach master.
I have a lot of blubber.
I am more agile in the sea than on land.
I asked the snail to walk a little faster because of the porpoise treading on my tail…
walrus

19. I give milk.
Trolls sometimes scare me.
We are Billy, Nanny and the kids.
My cheese makes a popular starter.
goat

20. I have big ears.
I eat 300 pounds of food a day.
I am the biggest land mammal.
Walt Disney called me 'Dumbo'.
elephant

6. My hide is thick and grey.
My horn is prized.
My horn is on my nose.
I live in Africa.
rhinoceros

7. I am a big cat.
I drag my prey up into a tree.
I cannot change my spots.
leopard

8. I live in China.
I am the emblem for WWF.
I eat bamboo.
I am black and white.
panda

9. I hunt at night.
I am the only flying mammal.
I sleep upside down.
Sometimes some of us eat fruit and others drink blood.
My big ears are used in echo-location.
bat

10. I roar.
I live in a pride.
The females hunt together.
The males have a mane.
lion

11. My home is called a sett.
I am known as 'Brock'.
I was a character in *Wind in the Willows*.
I have black and white markings.
badger

12. I use my tail as a prop when resting.
I have a pouch.
'Skippy' was my TV name.
I was one of Christopher Robin's chums.
I travel in large hops.
kangaroo

21. I am known as the ship of the desert.
I can take the hump.
My feet are adapted for walking on sand.
camel

22. I live only in Australia.
I am a member of the dog family.
I was falsely accused of a killing at Ayers Rock.
dingo

23. I come first in the dictionary.
I have a long snout and a sticky tongue.
I eat ants.
aardvark

24. I look very cuddly.
I eat eucalyptus leaves.
I carry my baby on my back.
koala bear

25. I have spots.
I am the fastest land animal.
I live in Africa.
I sound as if I don't play fair.
cheetah

26. I am close to humans.
PG Tips was my tipple.
I use tools.
chimpanzee

27. I can lose or make you money.
I am expensively trained.
Red Rum was one of us.
The Sport of Kings is associated with us.
racehorse

13. People sometimes think I am blind.
I can ruin your lawn.
I can dig quickly with my shovel-shaped paws.
The Jacobeans drink a toast to me (as the little gentleman in a velvet jacket).
mole

14. I roll up in a tight ball.
I am covered in prickles.
'Tiggiewinkles' is the name of my rescue centre.
I sleep through the winter.
hedgehog

15. I am very aggressive for my size.
I have a voracious appetite.
A nagging woman can be called after me.
I am Britain's smallest mammal.
shrew

28. I can live on country estates.
The autumn is the time we fight and bellow.
I grow new antlers every year.
Bambi was one of us.
deer

29. I have rust-coloured hair.
I sometimes raid the chicken coop.
My country name is 'Reynard'.
I was hunted on horseback.
fox

30. I have long ears.
I am mad in March.
I ran faster than the tortoise.
hare

3. Animal stars

(based on *Mental Aerobics* page 11)

Either give the name of the 'star' and ask the group to say who or what they were, *or* give the clues to the animal 'star' and ask for their identity.

1. Babar – King of the Elephants in the book by Jean de Brunhoff.
2. Moby Dick – large white sperm whale in Herman Melvilles's book (1851).
3. Paddington – a bear from darkest Peru, eats marmalade sandwiches.
4. Trigger – Roy Roger's horse.
5. Ferdinand – a bull who liked to smell flowers rather than fight.
6. Chip and Dale – Walt Disney chipmunks.
7. Garfield – comic-strip cat in the *Daily Express*.
8. Jumbo – world's most famous elephant, in Barnum's Circus.
9. Eeyore – sad, gloomy donkey in *Winnie the Pooh*.
10. Silver – the Lone Ranger's horse.
11. Cheetah – Tarzan's chimpanzee friend.
12. Mr Ed – the talking horse in the TV series.
13. Cowardly lion – in *The Wizard of Oz*.

14. Kanga and Roo – mother and son kangaroos in *Winnie the Pooh*.
15. Dumbo – Walt Disney's flying elephant.
16. Rudolph – Santa's red-nosed reindeer.
17. Nana – the Newfoundland dog in *Peter Pan*, who looked after the Darling children.
18. Thumper – the rabbit who befriended Bambi.
19. Rin-Tin-Tin – the German Shepherd who became a filmstar.
20. Jeremy Fisher – Beatrix Potter's fishing frog.
21. Elsa – the lioness rescued by Joy Adamson in Kenya, of *Born Free* fame.
22. Lassie – the collie dog who rescued everyone in the TV series.
23. Pluto – Mickey Mouse's dog with a silly grin.
24. Champion – the wonder horse.
25. Bugs Bunny – cartoon rabbit famous for saying 'What's up, Doc?'
26. Speedy Gonzales – a fast little mouse in a big sombrero.
27. Kermit – frog in *The Muppet Show*.
28. King Kong – 50 foot gorilla who terrorised New York in the film.
29. Snoopy – a beagle in the *Peanuts* comic strip.
30. Black Beauty – the horse in the story by Anna Sewell.
31. Heffalump – the imaginary large animal in *Winnie the Pooh*.
32. Lady – the pretty cocker spaniel loved by Tramp.
33. Bagheera – the black panther in *The Jungle Book*.
34. Sylvester – the cat who is always trying to eat Tweety Pie.
35. Booboo – Yogi Bear's little buddy.
36. Babe – the talking pig in the film of the same name.
37. Churchill – the nodding dog who sells insurance.
38. Scooby Doo – a dog who likes snacks but is scared of ghosts.

Add more of your own.

4. The parson's cat

All the group members in turn try to describe the parson's cat, each using a different adjective and all starting with the same letter. For example, the first person may say, 'The parson's cat is an **A**ngry cat.' The next person could say, 'The parson's cat is an **A**nxious cat'...'an **A**morous cat'...and so on, round the group.

In the next round the adjectives begin with **B**, and so on, through the alphabet.

5. Animal metaphors

(based on *More Mental Aerobics* page 104)

In turn, ask the clients to complete the metaphors.

as busy as a...bee
as sly as a...fox
as mad as a...March hare
as slow as a...tortoise
as blind as a...bat
as slow as a...snail
as sleek as a...cat
as tricky as a box of...monkeys
as fat as a...pig
as bold as a...lion
as free as a...bird
as hungry as a...horse
as weak as a...kitten
as quiet as a...mouse
as friendly as a...dog
as greedy as a...pig
as wise as an...owl
as stubborn as a...mule
as big as an...elephant
as proud as a...peacock
as strong as an...ox
as cold as a...fish
as tall as a...giraffe
as silly as a...goose

Ask the group for more examples.

6. Collective nouns for animals, birds and insects

(from *More Mental Aerobics* page 170)

Ask the group in turn what animal they associate with these groups.

1. school...*fish*
2. plague...*locusts*
3. covey...*partridge, quail*
4. army...*ants*
5. bed...*oysters*
6. den...*foxes, wolves*
7. pride...*lions*
8. pod...*whales, seals*
9. colony...*ants, beavers*
10. flight...*geese*
11. charm...*goldfinches*
12. pack...*dogs, wolves*
13. swarm...*bees*
14. brace...*pheasants*
15. litter...*kittens, puppies*
19. herd...*cattle, elephants*
20. brood...*chicks*
21. parliament...*owls*
22. ostentation...*peacocks*
23. leap...*leopards*
24. mob...*kangaroos*
25. warren...*rabbits*
26. flock...*sheep, geese*
27. skein...*geese*
28. murder...*crows*
29. field...*racehorses*
30. shrewdness...*apes*
31. chowder...*cats*
32. team...*horses*
33. sloth...*bears*

16. string...*racehorses, ponies*
17. poke...*oxen*
18. gaggle...*geese*

34. leash...*greyhounds*
35. crash...*rhinoceros*

Ask the group for more examples.

7. Animal quiz that gets harder

Ask members of the group in turn.

1. Which is the tallest mammal?...giraffe
2. Who is the king of the beasts?...lion
3. Puppy is to dog as tadpole is to...frog
4. How many legs has a spider?...eight
5. Name the largest living animal...whale
6. What is a flounder?...fish
7. Where is the scorpion's sting?...in its tail
8. What does a panda eat?...bamboo
9. When threatened what does a hedgehog do?...curls up in a ball
10. Where do kangaroos live?...Australia
11. What helps reindeer travel over snow?...wide hooves
12. What is the first animal in the dictionary?...aardvark
13. Name the largest member of the deer family...moose
14. Which camel has one hump?...dromedary
15. What is the organ of smell in the snake?...tongue
16. Where do tigers live?...India
17. If an animal sleeps through the winter, it is said to...hibernate
18. Which animals live on the Rock of Gibraltar?...barbary apes
19. What is the name given to mammals who carry their young in a pouch?...marsupial
20. Which is the fastest land animal?...cheetah
21. Name the only flying mammal...bat
22. Which mythical animal had a long, twisted horn in the middle of its head?...unicorn
23. Name the largest snake...anaconda
24. What is a gecko?...a lizard
25. In what is a horse measured?...hands
26. What are frogs and toads grouped as?...amphibians
27. How many species of shrew are there in Britain?...four: common, pygmy, water and Scilly

28. Are bats blind?...no
29. Which animal is featured on the symbol of the medical profession?...snake
30. What is the chameleon's special skill?...it can change colour to blend with its background
31. What are Charolais?...a French breed of cattle
32. How do millipedes protect themselves?...they give off an offensive smell
33. What is a basilisk?...a lizard
34. Which species of cat has cheek ruffs, tufted ears and a short tail?...lynx
35. Does anyone know the mythical creature on the badge of an occupational therapist? (Harry Potter's wand contained a feather from one!)...a phoenix

8. See how many words can be made from: ALL CREATURES GREAT AND SMALL.

Week 3 – Trafalgar Day (21 October)

Equipment: flipchart, paper, pens, paints or felt-tips to make signal flags, string. Nautical music, e.g. hornpipes, sea shanties. Copies of the 'Battleships' grid on page 207.

1. Reminiscence and discussion

Ask the group if they or anyone they know has served in the navy, either Royal or Merchant. What were conditions like? Have the sailors among the group visited any faraway places? Did they get a rum ration? Did they sail through any bad storms? Were they seasick? Anyone in the group been on a cruise? Is there anyone who has never been in a boat? Would *they* like to go on a cruise? Anyone dined at the captain's table? What was the food and entertainment like? Being in the navy in Nelson's time was very hard...but so was life in general in those days.

Because we are an island race we have a vivid seafaring history and many sayings and songs even today reflect this, e.g. 'Bottoms up', said when drinking, harks back to the time when the press gangs coerced drinkers in London's dockside to join the armed forces (usually the navy). Men who accepted 'the King's shilling' were deemed to have willingly contracted to join the navy, and one of the press ganger's techniques was to drop a shilling into the pint pot of a drunk or unsuspecting man, which would not be detected until the tankard was drained. The gangers claimed that the payment had been accepted and the victim was dragged away to spend what could be many years before the sail. Once the public houses became aware of the scam, they started serving beer in tankards with glass bottoms, and customers would be reminded to lift their pots and check for illicit shillings, with a cry of 'Bottoms up!' before drinking.

The 'recruits' worked long and hard, food was basic – meat salted in barrels, bread and hard tack biscuits – which often had weevils in them, causing many jokes about extra meat – and few if any vegetables, which gave rise to scurvy. (This was overcome in the late 1800s with the use of lemon juice, and strong recommendations to serve green vegetables with meat.) Drunkenness was prevalent – to numb the cold, pain and boredom. The men were issued *each day* with *one gallon of small beer* and *half a pint of rum*, which they mixed with water to make grog – this became known as 'Nelson's blood' after Trafalgar, when the great admiral's body was taken back to England in a barrel of rum to preserve it. This drinking led to many accidents and fights on board, which often ended with the men being flogged with the cat-o'-nine-tails, keelhauling, or worse. Women were not allowed on board – supposedly – but wives could come aboard whilst in port. However, the women who came aboard were usually prostitutes. Some wives did sail with officers and skilled workers. Children were born aboard – a boy of eight was the youngest person at the Battle of Trafalgar.

THE BATTLE OF TRAFALGAR, 21 OCTOBER 1805

The combined fleets of Spain and France were waiting in Cadiz harbour to take on the British Navy. This was to be the most important battle England had ever faced, as defeat would mean a clear way for a French invasion. It was a turning point in these islands' history – without Nelson, we could all be speaking French now!

The combined force planned to come out from harbour just off the cape of Trafalgar, in the usual battle formation of one long line of ships, towards the British fleet – whose normal response would be to form a similar line whilst they blasted at each other with cannon. Nelson formulated a different plan. He formed the fleet into two columns, one led by Collingwood, the other by himself. Nelson sailed his column at the centre of the combined fleet and Collingwood sailed towards the rear, thus cutting off the front part of the line. This caused a lot of confusion, as the combined enemy forces' ships had to manoeuvre back upon themselves to engage in battle. The British men were well trained and totally loyal to Nelson, they could fire three shots to one of the combined fleet.

Nelson must have had a premonition that he would die in this battle, as he spent the first part of the day saying farewell to his officers and asking them to be sure Emma and his daughter Horatia were looked after. (This did not happen, for they sank into poverty with Emma dying of drink.) Nelson then prepared his final signal to the whole fleet: 'England expects that every man will do his duty'.

Nelson wore his full regalia, in spite of warnings that he was making himself an obvious target, being in the thick of the action on the main deck. It was in this area that he was hit by a French sniper and died of his wound. His death dampened the sense of victory for the men, and they put Nelson's body in a barrel of rum to preserve it for his state funeral in England.

The death of Nelson caused immense national mourning, and his was the biggest state funeral given to a commoner, rivalled only by Sir Winston Churchill's in 1965.

The victory of Nelson over Bonaparte meant that England went on to become the ruler of the seas, never to be vanquished since that time, and sowing the seeds of the Empire. Ask the group if anyone has seen Nelson's Column. Where is it situated? (In Trafalgar Square.) The

V V
V V
V The British Fleet V
V in two columns V
V V
V V
V V

Λ Λ Λ Λ Λ Λ Λ Λ Λ Λ Λ Λ Λ

The Combined Spanish and French
Fleet in the more usual single row
battle formation.

Figure: The Battle of Trafalgar. Attacking in two columns as opposed to a single row reduced the targets and divided the Combined Fleet. The confusion caused and the fighting skill of the British sailors gave the British a famous victory.

column is 184 feet high, Nelson himself is 17 feet. Before the statue was erected the stonemasons held a dinner party at the top of the column, on the plinth. When it was cleaned in 2006 the cleaners did the same. The lions at the base were designed by Edwin Landseer and positioned in 1867.

It might be a nice activity for everyone in the group to make the signal flags on A4 paper and fly the 'England expects' part of the signal all week. (See page 206.)

2. Mimes

Conveying messages without words was essential in the battle. In this activity ask each member of the group to convey an activity to the others without words, by means of mime. In an envelope place a number of cards with activities written on them – one per person – such as ironing, shooting a rifle, batting at cricket, swimming, playing the piano/violin/guitar/banjo, telephoning, using TV remote control, driving a car, firing an arrow/dart, shuffling cards, etc. Each person has to pick one card and mime the activity.

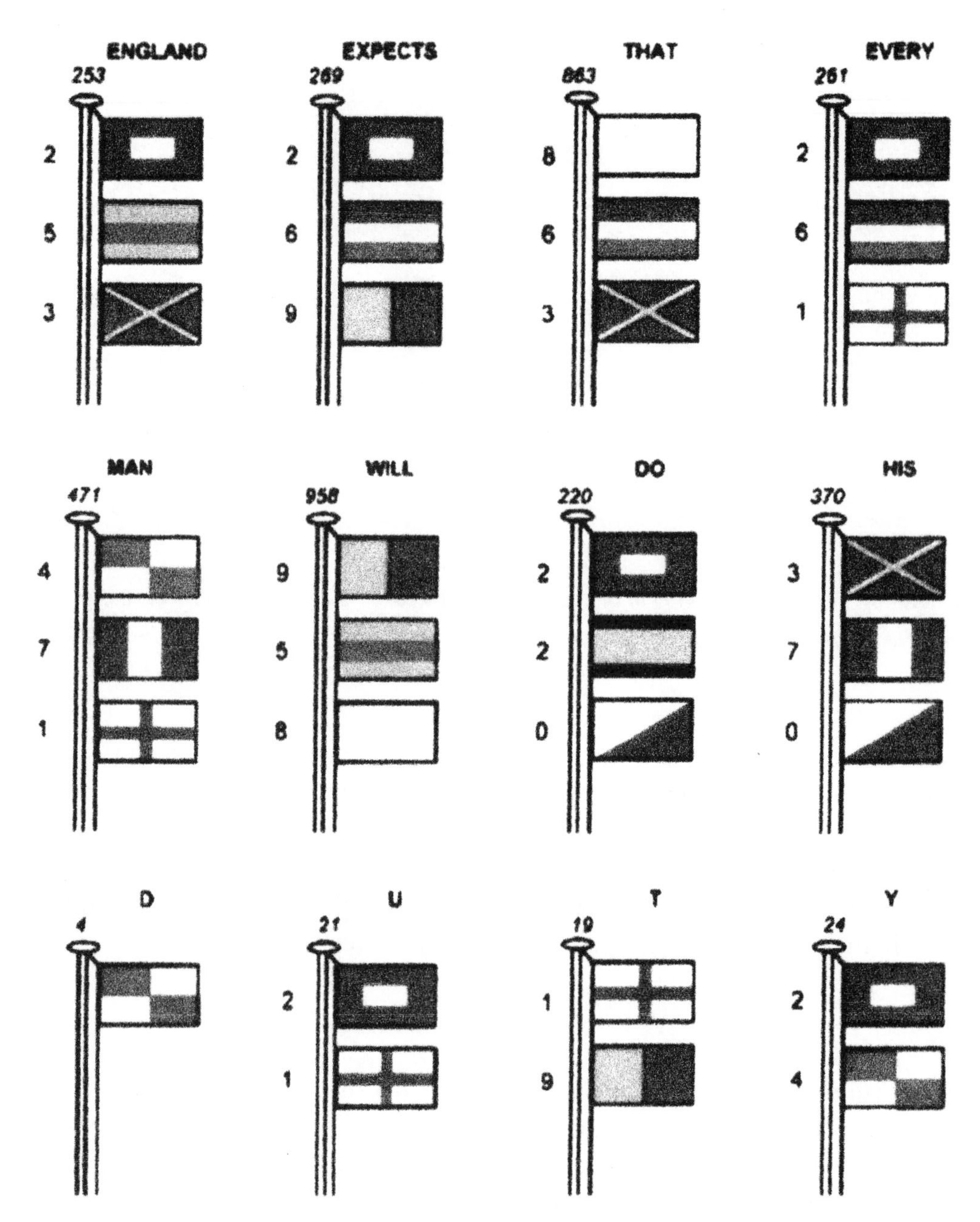

Colours of flags
0 = white/royal blue diagonals
1 = white background royal blue cross
2 = royal blue background white rectangle
3 = royal blue background yellow diagonal cross
4 = red then white upper rectangles/white then red lower rectangles
5 = yellow/red/yellow horizontal stripes
6 = royal blue/white/royal blue horizontal stripes
7 = royal blue/white/royal blue vertical stripes
8 = white
9 = yellow/royal blue vertical stipes

3. Battleships

In pairs, play a game of 'Battleships'.

Starting with a copy of the grid for each person, the players draw their ships over a grid by colouring in squares:

- 5 cruisers on each of 3 squares
- 3 destroyers on each of 4 squares
- 1 battleship on each of 5 squares.

Then in turns they pick a square (say, B8), and if their opponent has a ship on that square, he or she must admit to being hit – and be *honest*!

	A	B	C	D	E	F	G	H	I	J
1										
2										
3										
4										
5										
6										
7										
8										
9										
10										

4. Cat's cradle

Still playing in pairs, give each pair a piece of string tied in a loop, and see if they can remember how to play the old game of 'cat's cradle', which is like a reminder of the hammocks the sailors used on board.

5. Sea shanties

On the flipchart write the names of these sea shanties, explain their meanings and ask if the group can sing them. It may be best to write down one at a time and give its explanation. Shanties were used as work songs to keep spirits up and get a rhythm going for the task in hand.

Blow the Man Down

The 'blow' in this song meant the knocking down of a man with a fist, a belaying pin or capstan bar, not (as is often thought) the blowing of the wind in the sails. These were brutal times and the mates ruled with the fist and the officers with the cat-o'-nine-tails – a whip with nine leather thongs, often tipped with lead. Flogging was commonplace and death always close by.

Drunken sailor ('What shall we do with the drunken sailor?')

This was a work shanty used to help the men raise the anchor.

Fire down below

This was a pumping shanty to get a rhythm going to pump out the bilges, etc.

Holy Ground Once More

This is an Irish shanty about the 'Holy Ground' – the vice quarter near the docks of Cork or Queenstown.

Shenandoah

This was a windlass shanty sung when loading cargo from the dock to the hold. 'Shenandoah' was an American Indian chief in Missouri.

Hearts of Oak

The words of this shanty were by the actor David Garrick, who is also credited with the theatrical blessing 'Break a leg' – once he was so involved with acting a part that he failed to notice he had fractured his leg!

Dance to/for your Daddy

A Newcastle fishermen's folksong.

Anchors Aweigh

Surprisingly, this is about the army versus navy annual football match. There is fierce rivalry between the two armed forces even today.

Botany Bay

This is one of many songs written by convicts transported to Botany Bay for the least misdemeanour.

Bobbie Shaftoe

Is this song about a press-ganged lover? Very likely.

Nelson is reputed to have said 'One volunteer is worth ten pressed men.' How many other salty sayings can the group think of? For example:

- shipshape and Bristol fashion.
- to shoot a line. (Relates more to fishing than guns.)
- shove one's oar in.
- skylarking. (Refers to races in the rigging.)
- swinging the lead. (This refers to the sailor pretending to make a depth sounding, swinging the weighted line instead of dropping it into the sea.)
- POSH – 'Port Out, Starboard Home'. (The rich always had their cabins on the side of the ship facing away from the sun on voyages to and from the East.)

6. See how many words can be made from: SAILOR'S HORNPIPE.

Week 4 – Halloween

Equipment: flipchart, pens, local ghost stories (libraries or Tourist Information will have these), pumpkins.

NB Be sensitive to the feelings of the group. Some may not like to discuss Halloween for religious reasons, but most people will enjoy the fun.

1. Reminiscence and discussion

Explain the origins of Halloween to set the scene. Halloween has its origins in the old Celtic calendar. This calendar is very much based on the agricultural year and its first day was 1 November. The thirty-first of October was the eve of Samhain, the Lord of the Dead, and special rites and sacrifices were performed to appease him. The Celts worshipped the sun as the giver of life, and it would be growing less powerful, and the Earth beginning to cool, at the approach of winter. They believed that goblins, ghosts and demons roamed around in the cold dark nights, and they lit great fires to scare them away and so ensure that life would be renewed in the Earth when the winter season ended. The eve of Samhain's Day was celebrated with a massive harvest festival. This day was so important to the Celtic people, and their belief in appeasing the Lord of Death was so strong, that the early Christian Church could not eradicate it and so, because they were aware that the celebrations would continue, they re-dedicated 1 November to all the saints in heaven and it became All Saints' Day. The eve of that day became All Saints' Eve, or All Hallows' Eve, or Hallowmas, when special church services were held to protect the people from the Devil, the Evil One. Over time the name of this evening became shortened from Hallows Eve to Hallowe'en. The early attendants of Samhain's Eve still haunt the present-day celebrations of Halloween, with children dressing up as witches, goblins and ghosts. One explanation of the dressing up in scary costumes is that the ancient people thought they would confuse the evil spirits by dressing like them, and so not be seen as human.

Ask if the group can list some common Halloween symbols. Here are some, with explanations of their origins (from *Mental Aerobics* page 304).

- goblins: menacing, underground 'little people' or 'fairy folk' who could be evil and had some magical powers.
- witches: from the Saxon word *wica* meaning 'wise one'. Such people tried to understand the forces of nature, and this specialised knowledge made them appear to have magical powers.
- sorcerers: they also had extensive knowledge of the products of plants and animals – and they were able to use it to cure ills and to produce hallucinogenic states – to 'cast spells'. They kept their knowledge secret and made it more magical and occult.
- fire: this was used to scare away the evil spirits.
- black: the colour linked with Samhain, the Lord of Death – hence we have black cats and black magic. The shades of night and mystery.
- orange: the colour of the Harvest Moon, pumpkins and harvest.
- hex signs: used to scare away evil.
- salt and iron: witches would not touch these, so they were used for good luck.
- cat: cats used to be thought to have magical powers because of their stealth, night vision, light-reflecting eyes of yellow/green, and the way their hair stands so visibly on end at signs of alarm/threat. They were often the 'familiars' of witches. Even today a black cat crossing your path is thought to be unlucky in some areas.
- bat: parts of bats were found in witches' brews, and the witches daubed bats' blood on themselves. Because of this, and their sinister appearance and night flights, they became feared.
- owl: in ancient Rome these birds were thought to be the harbingers (bearers) of doom. Their glassy stare, soundless night flight and eerie call made them frightening.
- cauldron: a pot used to brew spells. Think of the three witches in *Macbeth*: 'Double, double, toil and trouble, fire burn and cauldron bubble.'
- ghosts: disembodied spirits of the dead were thought to return to their former homes on All Hallows' Eve, searching for warmth and comfort, or they were thought to come out of their graves and rattle their bones until dawn. Hence skulls and skeletons are symbols of Halloween.
- jack o' lanterns: strange lights seen over marshy areas. Sometimes lost people followed these lights further into the marsh and to their deaths. Rotting plants and animals in the marsh emit methane, which may spontaneously combust, causing

this phenomenon. Turnip and pumpkin lanterns are carried by children to scare away bogeymen and any other witches, ghosts or goblins that may be around.

- trick or treat: this is thought to be an American custom, but in fact it originally came from Europe where the practice of 'souling' took place on All Hallows' Eve as people went from village to village begging for 'soul cakes' – square bread pieces with currants. The more soul cakes they received, the more prayers they would say on behalf of the dead relatives of the donors, prayers that would speed up the transition to Heaven from the state of limbo that they entered on death. Earlier the practice was based on the folklore that there were demonic spirits wandering the countryside, frightening the villagers, who tried to placate them with food and fine treats to stop them destroying property and killing flocks.

Ask if any clients know a local ghost story, or select one from a your book. Did anyone make costumes for their children/grandchildren? What sort of games or tricks did they play on Halloween when they were young? Or were they not allowed to take part in this event because of religious feelings? Can anyone remember any TV series or films about ghosts or magic? (*Randall and Hopkirk Deceased*, *Bewitched*, *Casper*, *The Addams Family*, *Harry Potter*, *Ghostbusters*, *Buffy the Vampire Slayer*, etc.)

2. Halloween games

Make pumpkin lanterns. Can the group remember when they had to make turnip lanterns and how hard they were to carve? And the horrible smell of faintly roasting turnip when the candle was lit?

Apple bobbing will be too hard for many of the group, but staff may like to have a go and entertain the others. An alternative for the group is to have sugared, jammy doughnuts cut into halves and challenge them in turn to eat a half without licking their lips – almost impossible!

3. A Science and Nature quiz

Witches and sorcerers had great knowledge of nature – the 'scientists' of their day? Ask the group either in turn or as a general quiz.

1. What is the hardest stone?...diamond
2. How can you tell the age of a tree?...count the growth rings in the trunk
3. What is Britain's only poisonous snake?...adder/viper
4. What instrument lets you see minute particles clearly?...microscope
5. When a bee stings, what happens to the bee?...it dies
6. What is the chemical formula for water?...H_2O
7. Rosemary, sage and thyme are all what?...herbs
8. What makes a rainbow?...sun shining through raindrops
9. Name the forces of Nature that can drive a mill...water and wind

10. What is the scientific name for a tree that sheds its leaves?...deciduous
11. What turns litmus paper red?...acid
12. What is the chemical name for common salt?...sodium chloride
13. What do you call cultivated land?...arable
14. What are peacock, cabbage, comma and Red Admiral?...butterflies
15. What is the freezing point of water in Centigrade and Fahrenheit?...0°C, 32°F
16. Which is a conker tree?...a horse chestnut
17. The needle on a compass always points where?...north
18. Where are the seeds on a strawberry?...on its outside
19. What is the study of the weather?...meteorology
20. Whisky is not brewed, it is...distilled
21. What is the name of the Red Planet?...Mars
22. What is the process of food production in green plants using light?...photosynthesis
23. The stage between caterpillar and butterfly is known as...pupa/chrysalis
24. What is the study of shells?...conchology
25. A flesh eater is known as a...carnivore
26. What is the common name of the crane-fly?...daddy-long-legs
27. Which metal is liquid at room temperature?...mercury
28. What is the name of the single-celled animal?...amoeba
29. What is the toxic gas given off from an exhaust?...carbon monoxide
30. From which plant can you make rope?...hemp
31. Can you name a fly-eating plant?...Venus' flytrap, pitcher plant
32. What is royal jelly?...a rich substance made by the workers for the queen bee to eat
33. What is the chemical symbol for Potassium?...K
34. A wind blowing at more then 75mph is called...a hurricane.
35. An atom has three components. Can you name them?...proton, electron, neutron
36. What is the process of hardening rubber called?...vulcanisation
37. What is the study of fishes called?...ichthyology

4. Rhyming word game

(from *Mental Aerobics* page 120)

When making a spell witches often speak in rhyme. Read out each phrase and ask the group to give two rhyming words as the answer. Give Number 1 as an example.

1. excellent building material...good wood

16. digger's home...mole hole

2. old clothes receptacle...rag bag
3. sound slumber...deep sleep
4. inexpensive horn...cheap bleep
5. beagle's bark...hound sound
6. nude fruit...bare pear
7. inebriated animal...drunk skunk
8. inebriated insect...high fly
9. ordinary road...plain lane
10. happy boy...glad lad
11. perfect relief...pure cure
12. wooden limb...peg leg
13. dim light...low glow
14. audacious fish...daring herring
15. rodent's home...mouse house
17. arrogant drinking vessel...smug mug
18. level rug...flat mat
19. wobbly stomach...jelly belly
20. limping contest...lame game
21. dense bird...obtuse goose
22. odd ale...queer beer
23. humorous sweet stuff...funny honey
24. pressed cheddar...squeezed cheese
25. a woman of high fashion...slick chick
26. gleeful fruit...merry cherry
27. hooded bird...cowled owl
28. frightful airship...terrible dirigible
29. large archaeological site...big dig
30. fuel cavity...coal hole

5. Scrambled Halloween words

On the flipchart write the following anagrams. Give the group paper and pens to solve them individually.

GTSHO	ghost	OMNO	moon
TIWCH	witch	KISMORCOBT	broomstick
RACYS	scary	KNPPUMI	pumpkin
IONGBL	goblin	LJAEKONN'CTRA	Jack o' lantern
SNEOMRT	monster	OECSUTM	costume
WLO	owl	KPOSYO	spooky
TAC	cat	CTBEIWHDE	bewitched
RIITPS	spirit	WLOH	howl
VAERGDYRA	graveyard	WLOLENEHA	Halloween
LDUORNAC	cauldron	HCERSCE	screech
DBA	bad	NTHIG	night
VRAESHTONMO	Harvest Moon	TBA	bat
TROISUEYMS	mysterious	TEUHDANSHEOU	haunted house

6. Bible quiz

Because the day after Halloween is All Saints' Day it is appropriate to have a Bible quiz. Ask the group in general.

1. Who had a very colourful coat?...Joseph
2. What were the gifts of the Three Kings?...gold, frankincense, myrrh
3. Who killed Goliath?...David
4. Who was Samson's betraying lover?...Delilah
5. Who were Jesus' parents?...Joseph and Mary
6. What happened to Lot's wife?...she was turned into a pillar of salt
7. How many Commandments are there?...ten
8. Who betrayed Jesus?...Judas Iscariot
9. With what did Jesus feed the five thousand?...five loaves and two fishes
10. What did the dove bring back to the Ark?...an olive leaf
11. Where did the disciples fish?...the Sea of Galilee
12. Who asked for John the Baptist's head?...Herodias
13. How many are the tribes of Israel?...twelve
14. What was Jesus' first miracle?...he turned water into wine
15. 'It is easier for a camel to pass through the eye of an needle than...for a rich man to enter the Kingdom of Heaven.'
16. How many times did the Devil tempt Jesus?...three times
17. What was the miracle that Aaron showed the Pharaoh?...his rod became a serpent.
18. Who asked, 'Am I my brother's keeper?'...Cain
19. Where did the Queen who visited Solomon rule?...Sheba
20. Where was Moses given the Ten Commandments?...Mount Sinai
21. What is the shortest verse in the Bible?...'Jesus wept.'
22. Who dreamt of a ladder ascending to heaven?...Jacob
23. Where did Noah's Ark come to land?...Mount Ararat
24. How long did Jesus spend in the wilderness?...forty days and forty nights
25. What is the first book of the Bible?...Genesis
26. Who was called 'the Rock'?...Peter
27. To what did Saul change his name?...Paul
28. What language did Jesus speak?...Aramaic
29. Who was fed by ravens?...the prophet Elijah
30. Who doubted Jesus?...Thomas
31. What was the name of the chief priest who tried Jesus?...Caiaphas

Activities for November

Week 1 – Bonfire Night

Equipment: flipchart, pens, toffee (or fudge for people with dentures), parkin. Copies of word search grid on page 217.

1. Reminiscence and discussion

Ask group members if they celebrated Guy Fawke's Night when they were young. Did they have fireworks, did they build a bonfire? Can they remember guarding it on Mischief Night? (4 November was known as Mischief Night, especially in Yorkshire.) Was this tradition followed in their locality? This night was when children played naughty tricks on each other and neighbours, such as knocking on doors and running away, and the bigger boys used this time of mayhem to steal rivals' bonfires to add to their own. Did they have a Guy? How did they make it? Did they go round collecting a 'penny for the Guy' – and do they get asked nowadays for this? What do they think of the standard of today's efforts?

Does the group know who invented fireworks/gunpowder? (The Chinese.) The technical name for entertainment using fireworks is...pyrotechnics. These days this is a highly skilled activity, usually using a combination of music and exciting fireworks. Did everyone enjoy the fabulous New Year's Eve display in 2004 to mark the beginning of London's Olympic bid? Fireworks are made from saltpetre (potassium nitrate), charcoal and sulphur. (This is what gunpowder is made from.) Colour is given by the addition of various metal compounds.

Fireworks can save life when used as an SOS signal or flare at sea, or to light landing strips at night. Flares were shot into the air in the war and allowed to descend slowly by parachute to light whole areas. Smoke-producing fireworks were used for smokescreens to cover troop movements.

On the stage artificial smoke made from dry ice is used for scary, mystical atmospheres, or to add increased emotional atmosphere to the action, especially during musical concerts.

What do they think of the price of fireworks today? Can they remember what they paid? Did they have bonfire parties when their children were young? Who was in charge of the fireworks? Can anyone remember the Firework Code? Can they remember the names of their fireworks? (Roman candles, Catherine wheels, rockets, snowstorms, chrysthanthemum flowers, sparklers, cannons, bangers, jumping jacks or rickracks, etc.) Was anyone that dreadful boy who threw bangers at girls, who screamed in delight? Do they go to organised events now? Is this because they are safer? Or because of the exorbitant cost of fireworks? Should fireworks be banned from sale to the public and only allowed at organised events? Does everyone look after their pets especially well at this time? Any horror stories of this night?

Did they make special Bonfire Night foods? Toffee? Parkin? Baked potatoes? Did they bake them in the embers after the fire had died down – all black and charred on the outside and raw in the middle?

Can everyone remember the old rhyme chanted at this time? 'Remember, remember the fifth of November, gunpowder, treason and plot, I see no reason why gunpowder treason should ever be forgot.' Why do we celebrate this night?

In 1605, a group of Catholic dissidents, in an effort to force restoration of civil rights to the Catholic community, planned to blow up Parliament and King James I during the State Opening. The leader of the group was Robert Catesby and Guy Fawkes, a mercenary, was to light the fuse. At first they attempted a tunnel, but when that failed they secretly transported 36 barrels of gunpowder into the cellars of Westminster. The plot was foiled when a co-conspirator sent a warning letter to his relative saying that Parliament would receive a terrible blow on that day and those killed would not see who had done it to them. The authorities were alerted and the cellars searched where Guy Fawkes was discovered with fuses, gunpowder and a lantern. The conspirators were either shot trying to escape or were hung, drawn and quartered with Guy Fawkes after a short trial in January 1606. To celebrate his survival, James I ordered that the people of England should have a great bonfire on 5 November, and we have celebrated this ever since.

2. 'Fire' words

List all the words and phrases that contain the word 'fire'. Ask each person in turn.
Suggestions: fireman, fire alarm, fire engine, fire extinguisher, firecrest, fire insurance, fire blanket, fireproof, firewood, fireplace, Fire of London, firebreak, firefighter, fireball, fire irons, fire damp, forest fire, firefly, firelighter, firestorm.

3. Bonfire word search

Give everyone a copy of the grid on page 217.

J	U	M	P	I	N	G	K	L	A
A	L	B	A	N	G	E	R	J	P
C	G	U	Y	R	F	V	C	I	K
K	A	M	F	A	W	K	E	S	P
S	P	A	R	K	L	E	R	S	B
R	O	M	A	N	I	N	O	L	A
G	H	O	P	C	A	N	D	L	E
R	O	C	K	E	T	B	A	M	L
U	C	A	T	H	E	R	I	N	E
W	H	E	E	L	J	P	F	L	P

Can you find these words?

BANGER, ROCKET, GUY FAWKES, CATHERINE WHEEL, ROMAN CANDLE, SPARKLERS, JUMPING JACK

4. Right Royal quiz

(based on *Mental Aerobics* page 69)

Play in teams named after fireworks. Ask each team in turn.

1. Who was Prince Charles' first wife?...Lady Diana Spencer
2. What are his brothers called?...Andrew and Edward
3. Who was Princess Margaret's husband?...Anthony Armstrong-Jones
4. Who was Princess Diana's mother?...Mrs Shand-Kydd
5. What was the Queen Mother's first name?...Elizabeth
6. What was the Queen's nickname?...Lilibet

7. What is her London residence?...Buckingham Palace
8. What was the name of Queen Victoria's consort?...Albert
9. What is the Queen's favourite breed of dogs?...corgi
10. Where was King Arthur's Court?...Camelot
11. Where are the Crown Jewels kept?...Tower of London
12. Who guards them?...the Beefeaters
13. Which king was known as the Conqueror?...William
14. At which battle did he conquer England?...the Battle of Hastings
15. Who was allegedly our fattest monarch?...Henry VIII
16. Which queen had the shortest reign?...Lady Jane Grey
17. How long did she reign?...nine days
18. Which nursery rhyme is about Mary I?...'Mary, Mary, quite contrary'
19. Who is reputed to have removed all her mirrors when her beauty faded?...Elizabeth I
20. What event is held to celebrate the Queen's birthday?...Trooping the Colour
21. Which of the Queen's relatives was killed by an IRA bomb?...Earl Mountbatten
22. Name Princess Margaret's daughter...Lady Sarah Armstrong-Jones
23. What was the name of the Royal Yacht?...*Britannia*
24. Where are the monarchs crowned?...Westminster Abbey
25. What comprises the Crown Jewels?...sceptre, orb, crown, sword, coronation rings
26. What was the Queen's wartime job?...car maintenance
27. Who is her only daughter?...Princess Anne
28. What special title was she granted?...the Princess Royal
29. Who is next in line after Charles?...Prince William
30. What are Charles' other names?...Philip Arthur George
31. Who was Princess Anne's first husband?...Mark Phillips
32. Which Royal took part in the Olympics?...Princess Anne
33. In which event?...three-day event horse trials
34. Who was Prince Andrew's wife?...Sarah Ferguson
35. Who preceded Elizabeth II?...George VI
36. When did Elizabeth I reign?...1558–1603
37. What is Prince Philip's title?...Duke of Edinburgh
38. Where was the Queen when she heard of her father's death?...Kenya
39. What does the 'orb' signify?...the domination of Christianity over the world
40. Who was Prince Philip's great-great-grandmother?...Queen Victoria
41. When was the Queen married?...20 November 1947
42. Where are royal weddings held?...Westminster Abbey

43. Where is the royal Scottish holiday home?...Balmoral
44. Name Sarah and Andrew's children...Beatrice, Eugenie
45. Which race meeting does the Queen always attend?...Royal Ascot
46. What was Prince Andrew's nickname?...Randy Andy
47. What is Charles' favourite sport?...polo
48. Who did Edward VIII love?...Wallis Warfield Simpson
49. Who was Princess Margaret's first love?...Peter Townsend
50. Who was Princess Diana's grandmother?...Barbara Cartland
51. Which animals appear on the Royal Ensign?...lion and unicorn
52. What was Diana's job before she married?...kindergarten teacher

5. A quiz for history buffs

(based on *More Mental Aerobics* page 35)

This quiz could be done in blocks of 20 questions.

1. With which war was Florence Nightingale associated?...Crimean war
2. Which side of the American Civil War was led by Robert E. Lee?...Confederates
3. Which ship was allegedly unsinkable?...*Titanic*
4. Which attack by Japan brought the USA into WWII?...Pearl Harbor
5. Where is the British monarch crowned?...Westminster Abbey
6. In what year was Berlin reunified?...1991
7. Which President do we associate with Watergate?...Nixon
8. Where does Castro live?...Cuba
9. Who was the much married king of England?...Henry VIII
10. Who was exiled to Elba?...Napoleon
11. Who was the Polish leader of Solidarity?...Lech Walesa
12. Who was Queen Victoria's consort?...Albert
13. Who discovered the cure for polio?...William Salk
14. When was the Battle of Hastings fought?...1066
15. Who was the founder of the Vietnamese Communists?...Ho Chi Minh
16. Which fabulous aircraft flew first in 1969?...Concorde
17. Which sport is Eddie 'the Eagle' Edwards not so good at?...ski-jumping
18. Which Nazi committed suicide in Spandau in 1987?...Rudolf Hess
19. Who had a notorious affair with Christine Keeler?...John Profumo
20. Who sang 'Happy birthday' to Kennedy?...Marilyn Monroe
21. Which American song and dance man was born Daniel Samuel Kominsky?...Danny Kaye

22. Which world leader died in 1965?...Winston Churchill
23. Who wrote *The Little Red Book*?...Mao Tse-Tung
24. Which Russian ballet dancer defected to the West?...Rudolf Nureyev
25. The site of a nuclear accident in the Ukraine...Chernobyl
26. The flagship of Henry VIII's fleet...*Mary Rose*
27. Who was involved in the Gunpowder Plot?...Guy Fawkes
28. This concert raised 70 million dollars for Africa...Live Aid
29. What wooden contraption helped take Troy?...the Trojan Horse
30. In what year was Queen Elizabeth II crowned?...1953
31. What title did Hitler use?...Führer of the Third Reich
32. What name was given to the period of poverty, unemployment and social unrest in the 1930s?...the Depression
33. Who 'had a dream'?...Martin Luther King
34. Where did the Mau-Mau fight for freedom?...Kenya
35. Where was Franco head of state?...Spain
36. This young Jewish girl wrote a famous diary...Anne Frank
37. When did Edward VIII abdicate?...1936
38. Who was responsible for the Valentine's Day Massacre?...Al Capone
39. Who discovered penicillin?...Sir Alexander Fleming
40. How long did Queen Victoria reign?...63 years
41. Who created the communist state in Russia?...Lenin
42. What was Zimbabwe called before independence?...Rhodesia
43. What was the dance of the 'flappers'?...Charleston
44. Who founded the scouting movement?...Baden-Powell
45. What was the war between the British and Dutch settlers in Africa called?...the Boer War
46. Which American tycoon made a million by age 21?...J. Paul Getty
47. Who were two groups at war in 1993 in Yugoslavia?...Serbs, Croats
48. What was the drug that caused birth defects?...thalidomide
49. Which member of the Beatles was shot?...John Lennon
50. Who promoted 'glasnost'?...Gorbachev
51. Who was Prime Minister from 1957 to 1963?...Harold Macmillan
52. What did he famously tell the British public?...'You've never had it so good!'
53. Who was imprisoned on Robin Island?...Nelson Mandela
54. Who was killed at the Battle of Trafalgar?...Nelson
55. What was his first name?...Horatio
56. Which King was called 'the Lionheart'?...Richard I

57. In what year was the end of WWII?...1945
58. Who sailed in the *Mayflower*?...Pilgrim Fathers
59. Who was the first man on the moon?...Neil Armstrong
60. Who built the Pyramids?...Egyptians
61. In which year did Margaret Thatcher become Prime Minister?...1979
62. When was the Great Fire of London?...1666
63. Which country was known as Gaul?...France
64. What nationality was George I?...German
65. What was Nelson's ship called?...*HMS Victory*
66. What does the Bayeux Tapestry portray?...the Battle of Hastings
67. Which British King fought at Agincourt?...Henry V
68. When is American Independence Day?...4 July
69. Where was General Gordon killed?...Khartoum
70. Which queen ruled for nine days?...Lady Jane Grey
71. Who ended the slave trade?...William Wilberforce
72. Who urged the British to fight on the beaches?...Churchill
73. Who was the first American President?...George Washington
74. What were the Parliamentarians known as during the English Civil War?...Roundheads
75. Who did the Jacobites support?...the Stuarts
76. Who commanded the Eighth Army in North Africa?...Montgomery
77. Which Roman built a wall at the northern limit of the empire?...Hadrian
78. When did the Suez Canal open?...1869
79. Who was the first king to rule over both England and Scotland?...James I of England (James VI of Scotland)
80. When was the French Revolution?...1789–99

6. See how many words can be made from: CATHERINE WHEEL.

Week 2 – Remembrance Day

Equipment: flipchart, paper, pens, copies of codes (page 224) and the picture quiz (page 226). Poppies (NB If there are people in the group who have been adversely affected by the experience of war, or who have lost relatives, it is better to avoid any political discussion on the causes of war and to deal with the other facts of war, such as rationing, war work, fashions, music and comradeship.)

1. Reminiscence and discussion

Talk with the group about why we hold this day as special. Read this brief history to refresh memories.

Originally we set Remembrance Day aside to remember those who lost their lives in the wars of 1914–18 and 1939–45, but now we also remember those who died in the Falklands War and the wars in the Middle East.

Remembrance Day originated on 11 November 1918 at 11 o'clock (the eleventh hour of the eleventh day of the eleventh month) when peace was declared to end the hostilities of World War I. The next year, three minutes' silence was observed throughout the contending countries to remember those who lost their lives.

In 1920 on this day an unknown soldier was buried with full military honours at the Arc de Triomphe, Westminster Abbey and the Arlington Cemetery in Washington. In Westminster Abbey the plaque says: 'Beneath this stone rests the body of a British warrior of unknown name or rank, brought from France to lie amongst the most illustrious of the land... Thus are commemorated the many multitudes who died.' Since that time, each year at 11am on 11 November there is a two-minute silence, and wreaths are laid at war memorials. It has now become tradition that this day is celebrated on the Sunday nearest to 11 November to make observance easier.

Ask why we wear poppies as a mark of remembrance. (As a special reminder of the hundreds of poppies that flowered after the battle on Flanders Field.) At the Tattoo, during the sounding of the Last Post, from the ceiling fall thousands of poppy petals, one for each person who has died in conflict. People wear poppies with pride and volunteers collect money selling them for the British Legion.

a section from *Why Wear a Poppy?*
...our thanks, in giving, is oft delayed
Though our freedom was bought – and thousands paid.
And so, when you see a poppy worn
Let us reflect on the burden borne
By those who gave their all
When asked to answer their country's call
That we at home in peace might live.
Then wear a poppy – remember – and give.

by Don Crawford

Was anyone a member of the British Legion? The Legion was formed in 1921 by Earl Haigh to promote the welfare of serving and ex-servicemen. Its aim was to provide dignity and self-respect through employment, resettlement, rehabilitation and retraining. This is especially important for those who are disabled and their dependents, whom the Legion supports emotionally and financially. Seven million servicemen and women and nine million dependents are eligible for help from the Royal British Legion, so we all should wear our poppies with gratitude for their sacrifice.

Ask what branch of the Services people were in. Have they any relatives in the forces? Where were they stationed? What do they recall of those times at home or in the forces? (Only do this if it is not too emotionally charged.) Does anyone have any medals, wartime memorabilia such as ration books, demob cards, recipe books, postcards from abroad, uniforms, etc., that they may be willing to share with the group?

Did anyone parade on Remembrance Day? Was anyone in the Girl Guides, Scouts, Boys' Brigade, Girls' Brigade? Does anyone know a Chelsea Pensioner? How do you become one? (You have to have been a member of the Forces whose company saw action.) Was anyone a member of the Air Raid Warden Service? Or did they know anyone in it? What about the Home Guard? Was it like *Dad's Army*? What did they do? Any funny or horrific stories? Was anyone exempt from service? What tradesmen were exempt?

Can the group list – and sing – any of the hymns we associate with Remembrance Day?

Does anyone know any wartime poetry? Read one or both of the following:

In Flanders' Fields
In Flanders' Fields the poppies blow
Between the crosses row on row,
That mark our place; and in the sky
The larks, still bravely singing, fly
Scarce heard amid the guns below
We are the Dead. Short days ago
We lived, felt dawn, saw sunset glow
Loved and were loved, and now we lie
In Flanders' Fields.
Take up our quarrel with the foe;
To you from failing hands we throw
The torch, be yours to hold it high
If ye break faith with us who die
We shall not sleep, though poppies grow
In Flanders' Fields.

by John McCrae (a Canadian doctor/soldier)

High Flight
Oh, I have loosed the surly bonds of earth
Sunward I've climbed, and joined with tumbling mirth
The sun-split clouds – and done a hundred things
You have not dreamed of – wheeled and soared and swung
High in the sunlit silence
Hov'ring there
I've chased the shouting wind along
And flung my eager craft through footless halls of air
Up, up the long delirious burning blue
I've topped the windswept heights with easy grace

Where never lark nor eagle flew
And while with lifting mind I've trod
With high untrespassed sanctity of space
Reached out my hand and touched the face of God!

by John Gillespie Magee

Magee was a pilot who wrote this three months before his death in a mid-air collision.

Can anyone think of any war films they have seen? List them on the flipchart. Who starred in them? (Examples: *The Great Escape*, *The Colditz Story*, *Ice Cold in Alex*, *Sink the Bismark*, *Saving Private Ryan*.)

2. Code Breakers

In the war many lives were saved by the boffins at Bletchley Park who were our code-breakers and eventually cracked the Enigma Code. In November 2007 the very first computer (called Colossus) was rebuilt and tested against a German radio code transmission. All round the world computer buffs tried to beat it – during the war it took six days to crack the codes instead of six hours. Using the following code, see if the group can become code-breakers. Give everyone a copy of the code, or write it on the flipchart.

A	B	C	D	E	F	G	H	I	J	K	L	M	N	O	P	Q	R	S	T	U	V	W	X	Y	Z
1	2	3	4	5	6	7	8	9	10	11	12	13	14	15	16	17	18	19	20	21	22	23	24	25	26

23–5 8–15–16–5 25–15–21 8–1–22–5

We hope you have

5–14–10–15–25–5–4 25–15–21–18 4–1–25

enjoyed your day

1–20

at [insert code for the name of your establishment].

20–15 13–1–18–20–1 8–1–18–9

20–8–5 16–12–1–14–5 23–9–12–12 12–1–14–4 15–14 20–8–5
7–15–12–6 3–15–21–18–19–5 1–20 7:30 1–13
15–14 20–8–21–18–19–4–1–25 19–9–7–14–5–4
18–5–4 13–1–24

. . . .

20–8–5 18–5–19–9–19–20–1–14–3–5 23–9–12–12 2–12–15–23 21–16
20–8–5 2–1–19–5 20–15–13–15–18–18–15–23 1–20 7:0016–13

Make up more messages of your own. Ask the group to send messages to each other or the staff.

Answers: TO MARTA HARI THE PLANE WILL LAND ON THE GOLF COURSE AT 7.30AM ON THURSDAY SIGNED RED MAX; THE RESISTANCE WILL BLOW UP THE BASE TOMORROW AT 7.00PM

3. See how many words can be made from: BATTLE OF BRITAIN or REMEMBRANCE DAY.

4. Find the differences at GCHQ

Give everyone a copy of the picture quiz on page 226.

5. The great escape

Sometimes POWs escaped and used disguises. Can the group guess from the contents of these pieces of luggage what sort profession or interest these escapees were trying to portray?

1. Suitcase
- 10 blouses
- make-up
- 1 skirt
- contact lenses
- false nails and eyelashes
- 16 pairs of earrings

fashion model

2. Rucksack
- gloves
- blister cream
- suncream
- map
- 1 pair thick socks
- water bottle

hiker

3. Briefcase
- calculator
- laptop
- old school tie
- white shirt
- waistcoat
- files

city businessman

4. Trunk
- blazer
- name tapes
- ruler
- exercise book
- catapult
- video games

schoolboy boarder

5. Sports bag
- boots
- shin pads
- liniment
- shirt with number
- whistle
- pump

footballer

6. Sack
- spade
- fork
- muddy boots
- shears
- ball of string

gardener

Can the group suggest more?

6. Landmarks quiz

To fool possible invaders, the signposts were blanked out. Can the group guess where each of these locations is?

1. Northwest seaside resort with a tower...Blackpool
2. Where the Crown Jewels are kept...Tower of London
3. A stretch of water with a monster...Loch Ness
4. Where the PM lives...10 Downing Street
5. Where Nelson's Column is situated...Trafalgar Square

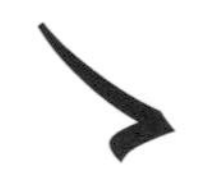

Answers: In right-hand picture: the birds are missing, chair back bigger, curtains patterned, ceiling light missing, picture added, seated man's shirt missing stripes, phone flex missing, pens in holder on desk, 'R' added to 'M' on name plate, fringe on mat under desk, woman's watch missing but she has a necklace, no braid on blouse sleeve, gate in doorway bigger, standing man's tie longer and mouth open, two extra dials on computer, waste bin by door

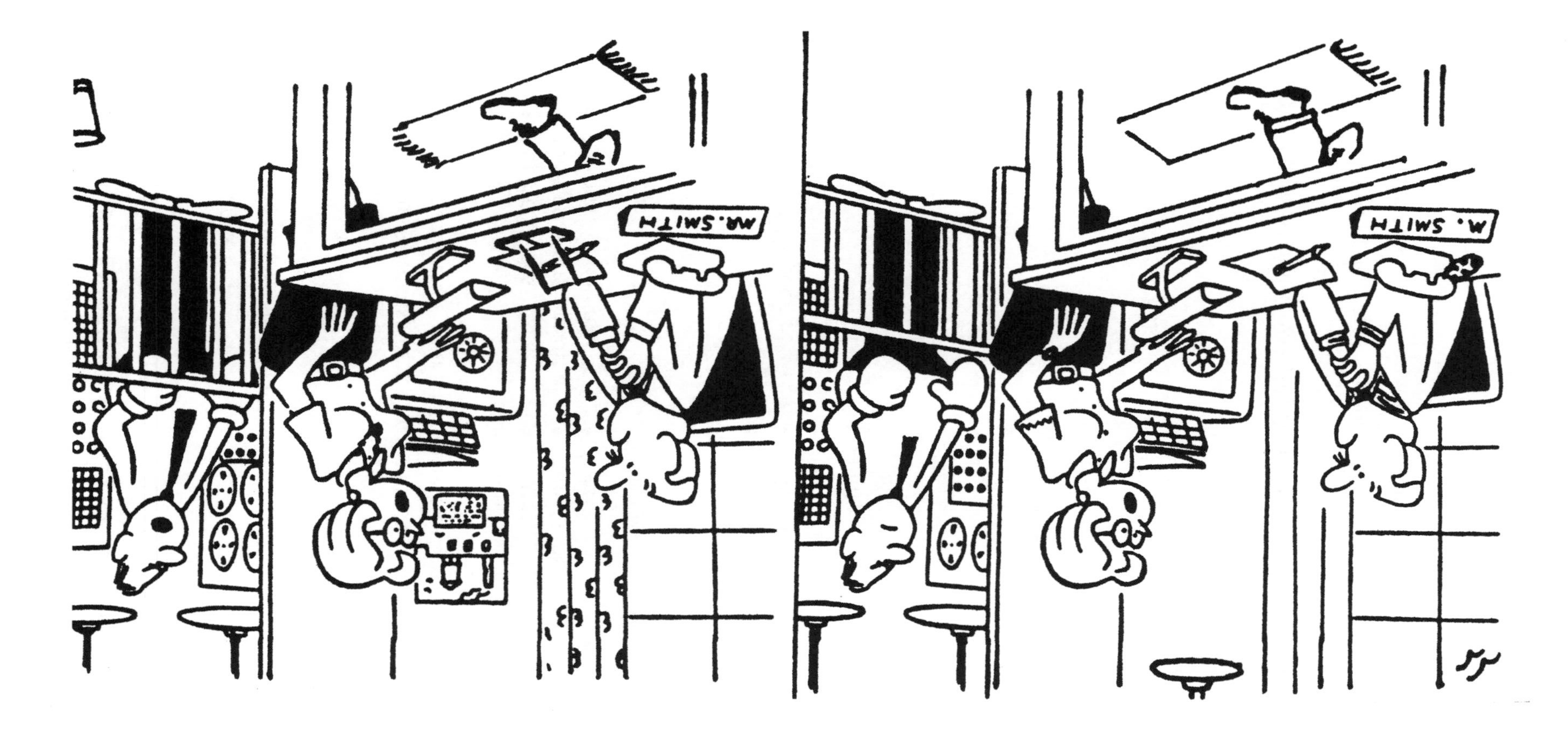

6. The Southwest corner of England...Land's End
7. The home of tailless cats...Isle of Man
8. The most famous university towns...Oxford and Cambridge
9. The London Bridge that opens...Tower Bridge
10. The London meat market...Smithfield
11. Where the blacksmith used to marry runaway couples...Gretna Green
12. The stretch of water in Norfolk...The Broads
13. Scottish Royal residence...Balmoral
14. Where the Crown Prince is invested...Caernarvon Castle
15. The Yorkshire County Cricket ground...Headingley
16. The stretch of water between England and the Isle of Wight...the Solent
17. Where are the Needles?...the Isle of Wight
18. What is the famous bridge at Bristol known as?...the Clifton Suspension Bridge
19. Birthplace of Lloyd George...Criccieth, North Wales
20. Birthplace of Shakespeare...Stratford-upon-Avon
21. The prehistoric monument on Salisbury plain...Stonehenge
22. With what did the Romans separate Scotland from England?...Hadrian's Wall
23. Where is the Liver Building?...Liverpool
24. The highest mountain in Britain...Ben Nevis
25. Where is The Shambles?...York
26. Where is Eros sited?...Piccadilly Circus
27. Which city is the 'city of a thousand trades'?...Birmingham
28. What is the largest lake in Britain?...Lough Neagh
29. Where are the Cuillin Hills?...Isle of Skye
30. Which city hosts the Miners' Gala?...Durham
31. Where is Poet's Corner?...Westminster Abbey
32. Where is Princes Street the main shopping area?...Edinburgh

Week 3 – Colours

Equipment: flipchart, paper, pens, copies of word search gird (page 232).

1. Reminiscence and discussion

Introduce the topic and then ask each member of the group their favourite colour – list on the flipchart. Ask what colour clothes they prefer to wear – has the colour of their school uniform had an influence on this? Did they wear a uniform for work? What colour was it? Ask if the colour they wear has an effect on their mood? (Bright colours = happy, drab or black colours = sad.) Has anyone made a mistake in the colour they have decorated their home? Or do they have a horror story about the decoration of a house they bought? Can people think of sayings using colours? (Red rag to a bull – by the way, a bull is colour-blind – white as a sheet, yellow-belly, green with envy, grey with pain, blue mood, in the pink, red herring, lucky black cat, yellow streak, etc.) Does the group know why we call special days 'red letter days'? Because on the calendar bank holidays are marked in red. Why do we wear black to a funeral? Is it true that Queen Victoria started this trend? (In fact she remained in mourning (black) for the rest of her life.) In some countries (e.g. China, Japan, Korea) their mourning colour is white.

Regiments wear certain colours – why? (So that they can identify each other from the enemy.) Some regiments wore red, why? (So the blood didn't show.) They use camouflage for protection. They troop their colours – what does this mean? (Parading their regimental flag.)

Cooks wear white in the kitchen – why? (To ensure that they change into a clean uniform when soiled.) Why do they use blue plasters? (So the plaster can be seen if it accidentally falls into food.)

What animals have a colour in their name? (Rainbow trout, Red Admiral, grey squirrel, bluestreak butterfly, cabbage white, red squirrel, Robin Redbreast, black and brown bears.) Some animals use warning colours, for example, wasps and bees, brightly coloured poisonous tree frogs. Some animals cheat by copying the warning colours when they aren't poisonous. Some animals use colourings to make them difficult to see, for example, tigers, leopards, lions, zebra, some bottom-dwelling fish such as plaice, etc.

Can the group remember the colours of the rainbow? '**R**ichard **O**f **Y**ork **G**ave **B**attle **I**n **V**ain' – red, orange, yellow, green, blue, indigo, violet – is a way of remembering (a mnemonic).

Coloured roses have special meanings. See if the group knows what they mean. Ask if anyone has received a very special bouquet. Would the men appreciate flowers being sent to them? Have they sent flowers with a special meaning?

- red = 'I love you'
- white = 'You're heavenly'
- pink = grace and gentility
- light pink = admiration or sympathy

- deep pink = 'Thank you'
- yellow = joy
- red and white combination = unity
- pale colours = friendship
- rosebuds = young at heart
- red rosebuds = pure and lovely
- white rosebuds = too young to love
- mass rosebuds = confessions of love
- single rose in full bloom = love
- bouquet in full bloom = gratitude

2. Personality and colour quiz

On the flipchart list the colours red, yellow, green, purple, brown, grey, blue and black.

Ask the group to write down their favourite colour, then put the rest in their order of preference. Read out the analysis and see if the group agrees.

ANALYSIS

Red represents passion and energy, as a first choice it means you are sexy, impulsive and like to win. You are a good leader and live life to the full. Red in seventh or eighth position of preference means your desire for life and adventure has diminished!

Yellow represents happiness and relaxation. In second, third or fourth place it means you are positive, optimistic and look to the future – never backwards. You find life easy, and have no problems. You lead a carefree life but you are not lazy, you can work extremely hard but not constantly. In first place it means you are ambitious, eager to please. If yellow is in the fifth to last position of your sequence, you have had your hopes and dreams dashed. You may feel isolated and disappointed, defensive and withdrawn.

Green represents firmness and resistance to change. Green in the first place indicates that you are persistent, possessive and quite selfish, a high achiever, an accumulator of things – penthouse, BMW, Rolex, foreign holiday home. You like to be recognised, and worry about failure. If green is a later choice you have had your ego bruised and your progression hindered, this could make you critical, sarcastic and stubborn.

Purple is a mixture of red, blue and violet and makes for a conflict between impulsiveness and calm sensitivity, dominance and submissiveness. People who prefer violet want a mystical, magical relationship, but may be mentally immature, dreamy and full of wishful thinking. Violet as a later choice indicates a person who has outgrown this fantasy vision of life.

Brown is the colour of physical well-being and indicates how healthy you think you are. In fourth or fifth place, this choice indicates that you are not very concerned with your health, so you are probably in good shape. Those worried about health place brown earlier in their sequence. As first choice it means you are restless and insecure; at eighth place it means you are not caring enough for yourself. Placing brown early indicates the importance of a secure environment.

Grey is a neutral colour between the opposite extremes of black and white. In first place it means you want to shut yourself off from everything and remain uncommitted, so that you can swing with emotions and opinions. You hate joining groups and prefer to observe rather than 'do'. In eighth place it means you like to join everything, are eager and enthusiastic and will try everything to achieve your goals.

Blue represents calmness and loyalty. High in the sequence it may mean you are sensitive and easily hurt, but you never panic and are in control of your life, and content with how it is going. You wish to have an uncomplicated, worry-free life and are prepared to sacrifice certain goals to achieve this. You want a stable relationship without conflict. You tend to put on weight – because you are so content? The later blue appears in your sequence, the more unsatisfied you are with life.

Black is a negation of colour meaning *no.* Anyone choosing black first – a rare event – is in revolt against their fate. As second choice, it means you are prepared to give up everything to achieve. In seventh or eighth place it represents control of one's destiny and a balanced outlook. If yellow precedes black in the first two positions, it means a change is on the way.

3. Colourful songs

Write the following songs on the flipchart (missing out the words in square brackets) and ask the group as a whole to find the missing word and sing the song.

1. [Red] sails in the sunset
2. [Green] grow the rushes-oh
3. [Yellow] rose of Texas
4. Two, two the lily [white] boys, clothed all in [green] oh
5. [Silver] threads amongst the [gold]
6. There is a [green] hill far away
7. When the [red], [red] robin, Comes bob, bob, bobbin'
8. John [Brown]'s body lies a mould'ring in the grave
9. She's as sweet as the heather, the bonnie [purple] heather
10. [Orange]s and [lemon]s...a hard one!
11. Three cheers for the [red], [white] and [blue]
12. [Blue] Moon

4. Find the colour

(based on *Language and Words Activities* page 35)

Give everyone a pencil and paper and ask them to write down the missing colour. Read out the following missing out the words in square brackets.

1. [White] Christmas
2. [Red] Riding Hood
3. [White] Cliffs of Dover
4. [Yellow] Brick Road
5. [Purple] Heart
6. How, now [Brown] cow
7. [Black] Death
8. [Blue] Danube
9. Heart of [Gold]
10. [Blue] Bird of Happiness
11. [Yellow] Submarine
12. [Green, green] Grass of Home
13. [Yellow] Rose of Texas
14. [Blue] Moon
15. Hurrah for the [Red, White and Blue]

Add more of your own.

5. Alphabet challenge

As a group go through the alphabet and see if you can find a colour for each letter.

For example: A – Aubergine, B – Blue, C – Cerise, and so on. Write them on the flipchart.

6. See how many words you can make from: MULTI-COLOURED SWAP SHOP.

7. Colourful word search

Y	E	L	L	O	W	L	E	Y	B
B	H	I	G	R	E	E	N	G	L
R	G	H	P	A	D	R	H	R	A
U	P	R	U	N	G	R	E	Y	C
S	L	E	M	G	A	U	V	E	K
T	S	U	R	E	D	A	Y	Q	U
A	L	I	S	O	L	I	M	E	N
B	R	O	W	N	T	R	U	O	C
M	A	G	E	N	T	A	A	I	R
B	L	U	E	S	I	E	G	L	O

Can you find the following colours?

YELLOW, RED, GREEN, ORANGE, LIME, BLACK, BROWN, BLUE, RUST, MAGENTA, GREY.

Week 4 – Famous men and women

Or adapt The Burns' Night theme as a theme for St Andrew's Day (30 November)

Equipment: flipchart, pens, paper, quizzes, collection of pictures of famous people (the picture quizzes from magazines, or pub quizzes, are very useful).

1. Reminiscence and discussion

Using the flipchart to list names, ask everyone to name at least one famous person who has made an impression on them – it could be a filmstar, TV personality, sports man or woman, actor, musician, notorious criminal, author, politician, inventor, historical figure, royalty – even a famous literary figure can be inspirational. They should say why their choice is famous. Ask if anyone (including staff members) has met a famous person, known a famous person, or maybe knew a person *before* they became famous. (Was there any indication they would be famous?) When they saw them, what were they like? Were they smaller/larger than they appeared on screen? How did they treat their 'public'? Did they believe in their own publicity? Were they surrounded by bodyguards or hangers-on? What makes these people famous – do they have a special quality? Did they have a special talent? What do people think about the celebrity cult we have at present? What are such people famous for? Will they still be remembered in the future, like those the group have listed?

Has anyone been influenced by the lives of famous people? Perhaps the bravery of someone inspired in times of trouble, or the tenacity of someone helped people to stick at a task. Would anyone like to be famous? For what? Could they handle the press and fans' intrusion, the vast sums of money? What is it like to be the child of a famous person? Can the group think of any who have suffered by being compared to their parents, or who have had such unnatural lives, because of the constant public scrutiny, that they couldn't cope?

2. Name that famous face

In two teams, each named after a famous person. Give each team a copy of your 'famous people' picture quiz and ask them to name as many as possible in 15 minutes.

3. Famous men quiz

Ask the group in general.

1. Who failed to blow up Parliament?...Guy Fawkes
2. Who was 'Ol' blue eyes'?...Frank Sinatra
3. Who had a famous round table?...King Arthur
4. Who led the Israelites out of Egypt?...Moses

5. Name The Beatles...John Lennon, Paul McCartney, George Harrison, Ringo Starr (Can anyone remember the fifth Beatle?...Pete Best.)
6. Who betrayed Jesus?...Judas Iscariot
7. Who said 'play it again, Sam'?...Humphrey Bogart
8. Who is the patron saint of Wales?...St David
9. Who was the first man on the moon?...Neil Armstrong
10. Who reigned in 1066?...William the Conqueror
11. Who composed 'The Messiah'?...Handel
12. What was Bing Crosby's nickname?...the Old Groaner
13. Who captained the *Golden Hind*?...Sir Francis Drake
14. Who founded the Scout movement?...Robert Baden-Powell
15. Watergate caused the downfall of...Richard Nixon
16. Name the Marx Brothers...Harpo, Groucho, Zeppo, Chico
17. Who was 'The King'?...Elvis Presley
18. Who said 'England expects every man to do his duty'?...Horatio Nelson
19. Which sport made Sir Donald Bradman famous?...cricket
20. Who was Satchmo?...Louis Armstrong
21. Who shouted 'Eureka'?...Archimedes
22. Who founded Methodism?...John Wesley
23. Who was murdered in Canterbury Cathedral?...Sir Thomas Beckett
24. Who first sailed single-handed around the world?...Sir Francis Chichester
25. Who invented the atomic bomb?...Robert J. Oppenheimer
26. Who brought in National Insurance?...David Lloyd George
27. How did Thomas Gainsborough become famous?...he was a painter
28. Who said 'Et tu, Brute'?...Julius Caesar
29. Who wrote *Great Expectations*?...Charles Dickens
30. Where did Shakespeare live?...Stratford-upon-Avon

4. Who am I?

(based on *More Mental Aerobics* page 98)

Ask the group to identify the famous women from the following clues. Give the first statement, then additional ones if needed.

1. I am the most famous blonde ever. I sang 'Happy Birthday, Mr President'. I still am an iconic sex symbol. My most famous picture was of me standing on a grid with my skirt blowing up. *Marilyn Monroe*

2. My mother was a famous singer/actress. She sang 'Somewhere over the Rainbow'. We both suffered from addictions and multiple marriages. *Liza Minnelli*
3. I am a cartoon figure. My boyfriend is in the navy. He knows eating your greens makes you strong. I am very thin, with a strange hairdo. *Olive Oyl*
4. I am a saucy actress from the 1940s. A life-saving device was named after me. 'Come up and see me sometime' was one of my many catchphrases. *Mae West*
5. I was the first woman. I was created from a rib. I enjoy fruit. Some of my friends are serpentine and duplicitous. *Eve*
6. I make lifelike models. I use a lot of wax. My first museum is in London. *Madame Tussaud*
7. I come from a famous Indian dynasty. I was the first woman prime minister of my country. I was assassinated whilst in office. *Indira Ghandi*
8. I am a woman in the Old Testament. A strong man loved me passionately. I was a sly hairdresser. *Delilah*
9. I am an Italian actress. I played opposite Peter Sellers. 'Goodness, Gracious Me' was one of our songs. *Sophia Loren*
10. I was Queen of France. I allegedly told my subjects to eat cake. I played at being a shepherdess. I met with Madame la Guillotine. *Marie Antoinette*
11. I was the most beautiful woman of the ancient world. My face was reputed to have launched a thousand ships. A wooden horse was involved in my life. *Helen of Troy*
12. I am the longest-reigning monarch. I wasn't often amused. I mourned my husband for the rest of my life. I enjoyed being at Balmoral with my ghilly John Brown. *Queen Victoria*
13. Love of me caused a constitutional crisis in the British monarchy. My first name sounds male. My prince showered me with jewels. We spent the rest of our lives abroad. *Wallis Simpson*
14. I am married to Johnny Dankworth. I am a jazz singer. I am named after an Egyptian princess. *Cleo Laine*
15. I have no regrets. I was a Parisian singer. My nickname was 'the little sparrow'. *Edith Piaf*
16. I led the fight for women's votes. Myself and my daughters were prepared to starve in jail. One of our number leapt in front of a racehorse. *Emmeline Pankhurst*
17. I was a famous opera singer. My great love was a Greek ship owner. I died tragically. *Maria Callas*
18. I wrote tales about animals. I lived in the Lake District. I was an expert on fungus. My characters are as popular today as when I first drew them. My books and characters have been made into a ballet, films, wallpaper, crockery, pottery figures and babyware. *Beatrix Potter*
19. I married the most powerful king of England. I was his second wife. He changed the religion of the country to marry me. I had an extra finger. I was beheaded. My daughter was known as the Virgin Queen. *Anne Boleyn*

20. I was an opera singer. I was a Dame. I had a dessert named after me. Peaches, cream and ice cream are the ingredients. *Nellie Melba*
21. I wrote many murder mysteries. I went missing in Harrogate. My play *The Mousetrap* is the longest running play ever. *Agatha Christie*
22. I was a famous dress designer. I was famous for the design of a jacket just after the war. My perfume range is very exclusive and expensive and was reputed to be all Marilyn Monroe wore in bed! *Coco Chanel*
23. I was an English actress. My roles included Queen Elizabeth I, films such as *Women in Love* and *A Touch of Class*. I am now a politician. *Glenda Jackson*
24. I lived on the moors in Yorkshire. I wrote fiction. My brother was called Branwell. My sisters were Charlotte and Anne. *Emily Brontë*
25. I was born in France. I was a peasant girl. I led an army. I was burnt at the stake. *Joan of Arc*
26. I was famous in the Sixties. I was a model. I was very slender. I was known by just my nickname. I now wear M&S clothes. *Twiggy*
27. I am American. I was born deaf and blind. I campaigned for improved teaching of the physically handicapped. A film was made of my life. *Helen Keller*
28. I was one of the first TV cooks. I bossed my husband around. He was called Johnnie. *Fanny Craddock*
29. I was a famous horsewoman. My long hair saved my blushes. I lived in Coventry. Peeping Tom tried to look at me in my naked state. *Lady Godiva*
30. My husband was a great wartime leader in WWII. I was a great support and influence for him. 'Oh, my darling' would give a clue to my first name. *Clementine Churchill*

Ask the group for more famous people, with clues to help the rest guess.

5. Who said that?

(based on *Mental Aerobics* page 85)

Match the names to these quotations of the famous.

1. 'Mad dogs and English men go out in the midday sun.' *Noel Coward*
2. 'Give us the tools and we finish the job.' *Winston Churchill*
3. 'The time has come, the walrus said, to talk of many things.' *Lewis Carroll*
4. 'Should auld acquaintance be forgot…' *Robbie Burns*
5. 'Come up and see me sometime.' *Mae West*
6. 'We are not amused.' *Queen Victoria*
7. 'Cauliflower is nothing but a cabbage with a college education.' *Mark Twain*
8. 'A horse! A horse! My kingdom for a horse.' *Richard II* in Shakespeare's play
9. 'Time for Bed.' *Zebedee* from *The Magic Roundabout*

10. 'An army marches on its stomach.' *Napoleon*
11. 'Hush, hush, whisper who dares…' *A. A. Milne* in *Christopher Robin*
12. 'If you can keep your head when all about are losing theirs…' *Rudyard Kipling*
13. 'Who will rid my of this turbulent priest?' *Henry II*
14. 'Let them eat cake.' *Marie Antoinette*
15. 'The quality of mercy is not strained.' *Shylock*, in Shakespeare's play *The Merchant of Venice*
16. 'Eureka!' *Archimedes*
17. 'One small step for man, one giant leap for mankind.' *Neil Armstrong*
18. 'Oh! to be in England now that April's there.' *John Masefield*
19. 'I must go down to the sea again, to the lonely sea and the sky.' *John Masefield*
20. 'A host of golden daffodils.' *William Wordsworth*
21. 'Half a league, half a league, half a league onward.' *Alfred Lord Tennyson* in *Charge of the Light Brigade*
22. 'To err is human, to forgive, divine.' *Alexander Pope*
23. 'Candy is dandy, But liquor is quicker!' *Ogden Nash*
24. 'England expects that every man will do his duty.' *Horatio Nelson*
25. 'Yabba Dabba Doo.' *Fred Flintstone*

Add more quotes of your own.

6. See how many words can be made from: FAME AND FORTUNE.

Activities for December

Week 1 – Favourite TV and radio shows

Equipment: flipchart, paper, pens, song sheets, prepared cards for '*Call my Bluff*'. It would be good to get a pianist to play the old songs for a singsong if you can.

1. Reminiscence and discussion

Using the flipchart, list all the songs on the radio that the group can remember from the war years. As a prompt, ask: Who was the Forces Sweetheart? (Vera Lynn.) What were her best known songs? Can the group sing them? ('White Cliffs of Dover', 'We'll meet again', 'When the lights come on again', 'Keep the Home Fires Burning', etc.) A singsong could be based on the listed songs. Ask for other old-time songs that were funny, such as, 'I'm a lonely little petunia in an onion patch', 'I'm a pink toothbrush'. Do they remember Uncle Mac who presented the children's radio request programme? What children's songs were played? ('Puff the Magic Dragon', 'The Runaway Train', 'The Quartermaster's Store', 'Incy Wincy Spider', 'There was an Old Woman who Swallowed a Fly', 'Y' Canna Shove y' Grannie off a Bus'.) Did everyone have a radio when they were little? Was it a mains or a battery one? Did they have to go and get new batteries each week? Anyone have a cats' whisker set?

What radio shows can the group remember? *Dick Barton Special Agent* – can anyone hum the theme tune? *Journey into Space* – can anyone remember what the Martians used to say? ('Orders shall be obeyed without question.') *The Navy Lark, ITMA* – what did the initials stand for? (*It's That Man Again.*) *Mrs Dale's Diary, The Archers* – still going strong. Can they hum the theme tune? *Round the Horn, Educating Archie* – does anyone think it strange there was a ventriloquist on radio? (Actually Peter Brough the ventriloquist was very poor, as you could see his lips moving all the time!) Can anyone remember the people who started out on this show? (Hattie Jacques, Tony Hancock, Max Bygraves, Beryl Reid were some.) *The Clitheroe Kid, Ray's a Laugh* with Ted Ray, Jimmy Edwards and *The Glums, The Goon Show* with Harry Secombe, Spike Milligan, Peter Sellers, Michael Bentine. *Family Favourites* was popular on Sunday mornings, connecting us with the forces abroad, as was *The Billy Cotton Band Show* – his catchphrase was? ('Wakey, wakey'.) *Top of the Form* was a popular inter-school quiz show –

did any of the schools nearby take part? Can they remember the theme tune? Wilfred Pickles and his wife Mabel took their show *Have a Go* round factories and workplaces. Violet Carson (Ena Sharples in another life) played the piano for them. Can the group remember the catchphrases? ('Give 'em the money, Barnie', 'What's on the table, Mabel?'and 'Good Neet'.) *Workers' Playtime* was a lunchtime variety show that also toured factories – did it go to one that any group members worked at? Does the group remember *Listen with Mother* and *Children's Hour*? Do they still listen to the radio? Which channel?

When did the group first get their televisions? Most people got one, or at least saw their first television at a neighbour's house, at the time of the Coronation in 1953. Does everyone remember the interludes between programmes – especially the potter's wheel? There was also a test card, which consisted of geometrical signs. What was the later one like? (A little girl with a clown doll, playing noughts and crosses.) Do they watch a lot of TV? What are their favourite shows? Can they remember when they got colour TV?

Do they remember the first police drama? – *Dixon of Dock Green.* What was his catchphrase? ('Evening, all'.) This was followed by American imports such as *Highway Patrol,* then our own *Z Cars* – can they hum the theme tune? The detectives we enjoyed were *Mark Saber* – the one-armed detective, *Maigret, Dragnet.* There were a lot of Western shows – *Gunsmoke, Wagon Train, Bonanza, Cheyenne, Rawhide, Maverick, Alias Smith and Jones.* Any others?

Light entertainment was provided by David Nixon, the conjuror, *The Perry Como Show, The Black-and-White Minstrels, Opportunity Knocks, What's my Line* – can the group remember who introduced this? (Gilbert Harding.) *Take your Pick, Sunday Night at the London Palladium.* Which topical show began with someone shouting 'Stop'? *In Town Tonight.* The presenter said, 'Once again we stop the roar of London's traffic to bring you...' and in the background there was a woman flowerseller saying, 'Violets, lovely violets.' *Come Dancing, Jukebox Jury, Cool for Cats, The Army Game, The Rag Trade, On the Buses, The Benny Hill Show, Upstairs, Downstairs, The Forsyte Saga...*

There were DIY shows such as *Bucknell's House* with Barry Bucknell, gardening with Percy Thrower, and one of the first TV chefs was Philip Harben.

The children had special entertainment with *Champion the Wonder Horse, Lassie, Skippy,* Prudence Kitten and Muffin the Mule, Johnny Morris with *Zoo Time,* fantastic dramas such as *Treasure Island,* and, for the little ones, *The Woodentops, Bill and Ben, The Clangers.*

2. Musical quiz

Read the following incorrect song titles one at a time, and ask the group to replace the wrong word in capital letters with the correct one (in brackets) and then sing the song.

1. My BODY lies over the ocean (bonnie)
2. If you were the only CURL in the world (girl)
3. There are GREY skies over, The white cliffs of Dover (blue)
4. There's no business like SLOW business (show)
5. FOOL, glorious FOOL (food)
6. We'll EAT again (meet)

7. Keep the COAL fires burning (home)
8. O what a beautiful EVENING (morning)
9. Thank Heaven for WALNUT WHIRLS (little girls)
10. I've grown accustomed to her NOSE (face)
11. There ain't nothing like a DRAIN (dame)
12. You are my HEARTH'S desire (heart's)
13. If I were a BIG man (rich)
14. A SUSSEX with a fringe on top (Surrey)
15. I know that my Redeemer GIVETH (liveth)
16. Climb every FOUNTAIN (mountain)
17. The corn is as high as an elephant's EAR (eye)
18. Singin' in the TRAIN (rain)
19. Sisters, sisters, there were never such BELOVED sisters (devoted)
20. Follow the ORANGE brick road (yellow)
21. A spoon full of TREACLE helps the medicine go down (sugar)
22. Wonderful, wonderful CONSTANTINOPLE (Copenhagen)

3. Call my bluff

You will need 30 pieces of card folded in half. On the *inside* of each, write the definition of a word on one half, and on the other half write in large letters whether it is 'TRUE' or 'FALSE'. Write the word on the flipchart, then have three members of staff – or three confident members of the group – read out the different definitions. The group is asked to agree which definition is true. The chosen definition is opened with great play to reveal the truth...

1. BALDRIC
   - True = A belt worn over the shoulder to hold a sword.
   - False = A lover of turnips.
   - False = An underfilled hayrick.
2. BOURDON
   - True = The bass drone of a bagpipe.
   - False = A type of chocolate biscuit.
   - False = Thick, fatty pieces of bacon.
3. AGELAST
   - True = One who never laughs.
   - False = A long lived person.
   - False = Made from gelatine.
4. ARACHIBUTYROPHOBIA
   - True = Fear of peanut butter.
   - False = Fear of yellow spiders.
   - False = Fear of toast racks.

5. JOOLA — True = A rope suspension bridge.
   False = A maker of gem stones.
   False = A kind of hula-hoop.
6. PECUNIOUS — True = Having a lot of money.
   False = A lover of pecan nuts.
   False = To pick at food.
7. THRIP — True = To snap one's fingers.
   False = A small, bloodsucking insect.
   False = The sound made by a cricket.
8. WUNTEE — True = A lonely, old, buffalo bull.
   False = An Indian washerwoman.
   False = A small tent made by North American Indians.
9. MALOPHILE — True = One who loves apples.
   False = A marshmallow lover.
   False = A kind of mellow coffee.
10. ZOB — True = A worthless person.
   False = A Norse god.
   False = A bulb of the shallot family.

4. What's my line?

With a little warning and time for thinking, ask the group in turn to mime a part of their pre-retirement job, or a household task if they did not go out to work. They should be visible to the whole group. The group then gets to make a guess at their occupation. Only allow three guesses before asking for a revelation.

5. TV programmes past and present

Read out the clues, write them on the flipchart or type them out without the answers and give a copy to each person, or group of three, to work by themselves. *For example*: The invoice = The Bill

1. Twelve months on the wall...*Calendar*
2. Magnificent platform...*Grandstand*
3. In the bedroom and in the lounge...*Upstairs, Downstairs*
4. Heavens after dark...*The Sky at Night*
5. Unlock academy...*Open University*
6. Celebrity journey: the subsequent era...*Star Trek: The Next Generation*
7. All those in the house next door...*Neighbours*

8. The enormous shatter-quick...*Big Breakfast*
9. Cruise and Lee-Lewis...*Tom and Jerry*
10. Creek Team...*Brookside*
11. Colour of mourning calculator...*Blackadder*
12. Resident and abroad...*Home and Away*
13. Every beast distinguished and diminutive...*All Creatures Great and Small*
14. Stop a taxi and tempo...*Hale and Pace*
15. Orient discontinuers...*Eastenders*
16. Twelve inches in the mausoleum...*One Foot In the Grave*
17. Land rehearsal...*A Country Practice*
18. Checker dots and dashes...*Inspector Morse*
19. Glance towards Scotland...*Look North*
20. Substandard skyscrapers...*Fawlty Towers*
21. Soaring surgeons...*Flying Doctors*
22. Interrogation duration...*Question Time*
23. Relics highway display...*Antiques Roadshow*
24. Summit of the fathers...*Top of the Pops*
25. Here is your existence...*This Is Your Life*
26. Appointment with Stevie Wonder...*Blind Date*
27. Obstruct smashers...*Blockbusters*
28. Wounded...*Casualty*
29. Send chap a gentle tap...*Postman Pat*
30. Manslaughter, the female transcribed...*Murder: She Wrote*
31. Desire your presence in my vicinity...*Wish You Were Here*
32. Firestick (a Lucifer or Swan Vesta) of 24 hours...*Match Of The Day*
33. Remnants of the hot season plonk...*Last Of The Summer Wine*
34. Does not shut for a minute...*Open All Hours*
35. Wrongdoing chronometer...*Crimewatch*
36. Pornographic Ustinov...*Blue Peter*
37. Adore ecstasy...*Lovejoy*
38. Small rock factory...*Pebble Mill*
39. Chinese royal regime...*Dynasty*
40. Marijuana opposite to white...*Pot Black*

6. See how many words can be made from: THE RADIO TIMES.

Week 2 – The local flea pit or going to the cinema

Equipment: flipchart, pens, quizzes.

1. Reminiscence and discussion

Talk about the films the group saw in their youth. Do they all recall the same ones? Does anyone remember seeing the earliest talkies? Ask each person their favourite film, what it was about and why it especially touched them. What was the first film they saw? How old were they? What was the name of the cinema they went to? Do they call the films 'movies', 'pictures' or 'flicks'? Did they go to the Saturday matinee? Which seats did they sit in? Was there other entertainment on at the same time? Can anyone remember the names of the heroes they watched? (Batman, Superman, Tarzan, Nyoka the Jungle Girl, Roy Rogers, The Cisco Kid, Hopalong Cassidy.) Did they run home with their coats fastened round their necks as a cloak, or did they 'ride' home on an imaginary horse, making 'clippety-clop' noises and with a switchy stick smacking their own behind, and shooting with their fingers?

Did their cinema have an electric organ that went up and down? Did they sing along to a film with the words of the song, like a subtitle and a bouncy ball, hitting each word in time? When they were first courting did they go to the cinema to sit in the dark on the back row? Was there an interval in the film when they could buy icecream? What else was sold to eat whilst watching the film? Did they buy their sweetheart a box of chocolates or Paynes Poppets before they went into the cinema? Were they shown to their seat by an usherette with a torch? What was the name of the news film? (Pathe.) What was the symbol shown? (A crowing cockerel.) For the price of a ticket did they usually get a cartoon, the news and the main feature? Can anyone name any famous film studios? (Warner Bros, Walt Disney, Rank, Pinewood, Hammer, Elstree.)

On the flipchart, ask the group to list as many filmstars as they can. It may be interesting to set a figure to attain (or for services users on other days to beat).

Does anyone still go to the cinema, or do they hire a video or DVD, or just watch films on TV? Do they feel it is more atmospheric to watch a film with an audience in a darkened cinema? Do they think they would go if they had someone to go with? Maybe this could be used as a link-up. OAPs get concessions at the cinema, and showings are held in the afternoon. Or maybe the group could choose a video to watch together at the centre/in the TV lounge.

What do they think about modern cinema? Are they impressed with the special effects? Which modern film have they enjoyed, or would like to see?

2. Animal stars

(based on *Mental Aerobics* page 11)

Does anyone remember any films with animals as stars? The answers to the following are the names of animal characters in films, stories or cartoons. Ask the group in general.

1. The king of the Elephants in the story by Jean de Brunhoff...Bar bar
2. The hunted white sperm whale...Moby Dick
3. A bear who keeps marmalade sandwiches under his hat...Paddington
4. Roy Roger's horse...Trigger
5. The gentle bull who liked to sniff the flowers...Ferdinand
6. Disney's naughty chipmunks...Chip 'n Dale
7. A fat cat in a strip cartoon...Garfield
8. Famous elephant from Barnum's Circus...Jumbo
9. The sad, gloomy friend of Pooh...Eeyore
10. And his antipodean mother-and-son chums...Kanga and Roo
11. The Lone Ranger's horse...Silver
12. Tarzan's chimpanzee companion...Cheetah
13. The talking horse on television...Mr Ed
14. The feline in *The Wizard of Oz*...the Cowardly Lion
15. The flying elephant...Dumbo
16. Santa's red-nosed helpmate...Rudolph
17. The dog in Peter Pan...Nana
18. Thumper's friend...Bambi
19. German shepherd dog of TV and movie fame...Rin-Tin-Tin
20. Joy Adamson's famous lioness...Elsa
21. The villainous cat in Cinderella...Lucifer
22. The most famous collie in the world...Lassie
23. A talking white mouse...Stuart Little
24. Mickey Mouse's dog...Pluto
25. The wise old animal in *The Wind in the Willows*...Badger
26. The wonder horse...Champion
27. Warner Bros little mouse with a big sombrero...Speedy Gonzales
28. The three goats who wished to cross a bridge...Billygoats Gruff
29. 'What's up, Doc?' is his catchphrase...Bugs Bunny
30. Anna Sewell's equine hero...Black Beauty
31. The giant gorilla who terrorised New York...King Kong
32. The beagle in 'Peanuts'...Snoopy
33. Tramp's beloved...Lady
34. Pinocchio's moral friend...Jiminy Cricket
35. Who tries to capture Tweety Pie?...Sylvester
36. The black panther in *The Jungle Book*...Bagheera

37. The frog star of *The Muppet Show*...Kermit
38. The imaginary animal in *Winnie the Pooh*...Heffalump
39. Beatrix Potter's hedgehog washerwoman...Mrs Tiggy-Winkle
40. The fat rat who wanted Tom Kitten in a pudding...Samuel Whiskers
41. A talking pig...Babe
42. A little mouse who is adopted by a family...Stuart Little
43. A long-suffering dog who looks after Wallace...Gromit
44. Annette Mills' stringy sidekick...Muffin the Mule
45. A bear with a red jumper...Rupert

Ask the group/staff to add more of their favourites.

3. Films of the Thirties to the Eighties

(from *More Mental Aerobics* page 71)

Ask the group to fill in the missing word from each film title. Read them out, minus the bracketed word/s. Can they name any of the stars?

1. The Wizard of [Oz]
2. The Adventures of [Mark] Twain
3. The [African] Queen
4. [King] Kong
5. For Whom [the Bell Tolls]
6. [Forty-second] Street
7. The [Thin] Man
8. [The] Adventures of Robin [Hood]
9. Around [the World] in 80 [Days]
10. [Arsenic] and Old [Lace]
11. Guys and [Dolls]
12. High [Noon]
13. The [Inn] of the Sixth [Happiness]
14. Anchors [Away]
15. [The] Bridge on the [River Kwai]
16. [Bus]Stop
24. Death of a [Salesman]
25. Calamity [Jane]
26. From [Here] to Eternity
27. Gentlemen [Prefer] Blondes
28. [Bonnie] and Clyde
29. Some [Like it] Hot
30. Gone [with] the [Wind]
31. Born [Free]
32. [Butch] Cassidy and the [Sundance] Kid
33. Close [Encounters] of the [Third] Kind
34. E.[T.]
35. The Eagle has [Landed]
36. Easy [Rider]
37. The [Empire] Strikes Back
38. Guess [Who's] Coming [to Dinner]
39. Indiana [Jones] and the Temple [of Doom]

17. The [Caine] Mutiny
18. [How Green] was My Valley
19. Good-bye [Mr Chips]
20. Jane [Eyre]
21. Citizen [Kane]
22. [Double] Indemnity
23. [A] Farewell [to] Arms
40. [Crocodile] Dundee
41. [The] Sting
42. [Zorba] the Greek
43. [An] Officer [and a] Gentleman
44. The [Great] Gatsby
45. [In] the Heat of the [Night]

Ask the group and staff to add more of their own.

4. See how many words can be made from: THE ODEON CINEMA.

Week 3 – Musicals and panto

Equipment: flipchart, paper, pens, programmes and flyers from local theatre, records of songs from the shows, copies of word search gird on page 249.

1. Reminiscence and discussion

At this time of year lots of people visit the theatre to see either a pantomime or a musical. Can the group remember doing this when they were small? Or did they take their own children/grandchildren? Make a list on the flipchart of all the pantomimes the group can remember. Did anyone perform in a pantomime as part of their local amateur drama group? Did anything funny/disastrous happen? Does the group prefer the local am-dram pantomime to the glossy professional ones? Who is starring in the local one? Show publicity/ programmes obtained from the local theatre. Sometimes the cast will visit and do a song or two for residents. Does the group dislike the way that pantomimes are written now, with all the B-list celebrities starring? How do they feel about the way the scripts are written, with innuendo and sexually explicit references? Has anyone – group member or staff – ever written a pantomime script? Would they like to write one for the centre/house – with assistance, of course, and maybe put it on in January?

Does the group enjoy musicals? Which ones have they seen, on either stage or screen? Make a list. Musicals have been part of the English stage for many years – *Oklahoma* and *Annie Get Your Gun* opened in 1948. Ask if anyone can remember a song from each one they list? Can they sing or hum the tune? Can they remember who starred in the musical? Andrew Lloyd Webber and Tim Rice have been responsible for a great upsurge in English musicals – has the group seen any of them? What does the group think of the folk who go many times to see the same show, often dressed in character – shows such as *Joseph and the Amazing Technicol-*

our Dreamcoat and *The Sound of Music*? Has anyone present done this? Have any of the group's children/grandchildren been in a show at school – for example, *Bugsy Malone*? Which part of the musical does the group enjoy – song or dance? Who do they think is the best 'hoofer' – Fred Astaire, Danny Kaye or Gene Kelly?

2. Name that tune

Using the CD/record of the shows, play the start of a tune and see if the group can name it and the show it came from.

3. 'Oh no! It isn't' quiz

Ask the group in general:

1. Who is Widow Twanky's son?...Aladdin
2. What did the Fairy Godmother need to make Cinderella's coach?...a pumpkin and six white mice
3. What did the giant at the top of the beanstalk say?...'Fee, fi, fo, fum, I smell the blood of an Englishman. Be he alive or be he dead, I'll grind his bones to make my bread.'
4. What did the clever cat wear?...Boots
5. Name the Seven Dwarves...Sleepy, Dopey, Doc, Happy, Grumpy, Bashful, Sneezy
6. From what was the witch's house made in *Babes in the Wood*?...Gingerbread
7. What did Jack get in exchange for the cow?...three magic beans
8. What did the Evil Queen ask her mirror?...'Mirror, mirror on the wall, Who's the fairest of us all?'
9. How did Prince Charming find Cinderella again?...by trying her lost glass slipper on every girl in his kingdom
10. [*Have the group shout out the answer.*] What warning of impending doom is always given in every pantomime?...BEHIND YOU!

4. Music and songs quiz

(based on *More Mental Aerobics* page 75)

This could be done as a group or team activity with pen and paper.

1. Name four wind instruments...clarinet, flute, trumpet, bassoon, saxophone, recorder, oboe, trombone
2. Name four percussion instruments...drum, cymbal, piano, xylophone, triangle, bells
3. What are the musical sounds expressed on paper called?...notes
4. What is the note in the middle of the piano called?...Middle C
5. Who wrote the Blue Danube?...Strauss

6. Who composed *Aida*?...Verdi
7. Which famous piece is often performed as a ballet at Christmas time?...*The Nutcracker Suite*
8. What does Debussy's 'Clair de lune' translate into?...*Light of the Moon*
9. Who was Old Satchmo?...Louis Armstrong
10. Which hymn became a popular song in the seventies, played by a pipe band?...'Amazing Grace'
11. How many songs can you name with these colours in the title?
    - Red...Red Sails in the Sunset, Red Roses for a Blue Lady, Red Red Robin
    - Yellow...Yellow Rose of Texas, Tie a Yellow Ribbon, Yellow Submarine
    - Blue...Blue Skies, Blue Suede Shoes, My Blue Heaven, Blue Moon, Blue Christmas, Blue Hawaii
    - Black...Bye Bye Blackbird, That Old Black Magic
    - Green...Greensleeves, Green, Green Grass of Home
    - White...I'm Dreaming of a White Christmas, White Cliffs of Dover
    - Brown...Little Brown Jug, John Brown's Body, Don't Make my Brown Eyes Blue
12. Many people think this is the Australian National Anthem...'Waltzing Matilda'
13. What was Marlene Dietrich's famous wartime song?...'Lilli Marlene'
14. Who wrote *The Pirates of Penzance*?...Gilbert and Sullivan
15. Ask the group to sing the first line of the following songs, or *you* say or sing the first line, and ask for the title.

Title	*First line*
The Band Played On	Casey would waltz with the strawberry blonde.
Five Foot Two	Five foot two, eyes of blue.
Side By Side	Oh, we ain't got a barrel of money.
Diane	I'm in heaven when I see your smile.
Little Brown Jug	My wife and I live all alone.
Bicycle Made For Two	Daisy, Daisy, give me your answer do.
O, Susannah	I came from Alabama with a banjo on my knee.

Add more of your own.

5. Word search

S	T	O	R	Y	P	Q	T	N	W
A	S	P	E	C	T	S	H	E	E
A	T	I	V	E	L	T	G	V	A
S	N	O	W	K	M	O	I	O	C
C	I	N	D	E	R	E	L	L	A
G	W	H	I	T	E	Y	R	P	T
S	S	E	R	P	X	E	A	W	S
I	O	S	B	E	C	A	T	E	X
D	F	S	O	U	T	H	S	S	A
E	P	A	C	I	F	I	C	T	E

Can you find the following shows and pantomimes?

EVITA, CATS, CINDERELLA, SOUTH PACIFIC, STARLIGHT EXPRESS, ASPECTS OF LOVE, WEST SIDE STORY, SNOW WHITE

6. See how many words can be found in: THE UGLY SISTERS.

Week 4 – Christmas time

This week is for your own traditional festivities, decorating trees/rooms, making Christmas cards, singing carols, present wrapping, and traditional family games such as Charades and 'Guess Who?', 'What am I?'

- Out of their hearing, a selected person is given the name of a famous person, real or fictitious, or a seasonal item such as 'Christmas Pudding'. They have 20 attempts to guess their name, with questions being answered by 'yes' or 'no'.
- Try to organise a visit from the local Church, primary school or choir to sing carols. Printed songsheets will help folk join in.
- Sometimes the local school will enjoy coming to perform their Nativity Play.

Week 5 – New Year and calendars

Equipment: flipchart, paper, pens, quizzes, video of *Calendar Girls.*

1. Reminiscence and discussion

Talk about New Year traditions, which go back hundreds of years. Ask the group how they celebrated the New Year. Do they still follow the old traditions? Why is this time significant to people? (It is like a chance to have a fresh start, a way of drawing a line under what may have been a bad year and hoping for a better time next year.) The month of January takes its name from the god Janus, the two-headed god of gateways and doors, illustrating the closing of the old year and the opening of a new one. It is not celebrated at the same time for all. The Jewish New Year is called Rosh Hashanah and is celebrated in September, and the Chinese celebrate New Year (their most important holiday) on 12 February. In Scotland they make more of the New Year or Hogmanay than Christmas, sometimes giving their children presents at this time rather than on Christmas Day.

What does the group feel about the way we have come to celebrate New Year in England, with fireworks and first-footing? Do people make New Year resolutions? On the flipchart make a list of everyone's (including staff) resolutions. Do they never make them, as they know they will be unable to keep them? If they have made them, which one have they managed to keep the longest?

Ask how people envisage the 'shape' of a year – do they see it as a circle with seasons, like a clockface with summer at the top, autumn halfway round, then winter leading up to spring? or is it a straight line? Where does their year start and end? Some start in September, like the school new intake, some in spring or winter.

Does everyone have a calendar? What type? Do they use it as a diary? What kind of pictures do they like on their calendars? How do people remember how many days there are in each month? Do they use the old mnemonic 'Thirty days hath September, April, June and November, all the rest have thirty-one, excepting February alone, which has twenty-eight days clear, but twenty-nine in each leap year'? Why do we have a leap year? (Because the earth takes 365 days *and six hours* to orbit the sun, so every four years we get an extra day to keep the calendar in time with the sun. What can a woman traditionally do in a leap year? (Propose.) Has anyone in the group taken advantage of this tradition? Has anyone seen the film *Calendar Girls*? What does the group think of all the nude calendars that different groups of people have made to raise money since this film? Would any of them dream of doing such a thing? Would they like to see the film?

The days of the week are named after ancient gods. Which is the only day named after a Roman god? (Saturday, after Saturn.) Did the group members used to do certain tasks on certain days of the week? Can they remember them? (Wash on a Monday, iron on a Tuesday, etc.) Do they still feel they have to do this? What about spring-cleaning – do they still do this, or is it unnecessary with all the modern appliances keeping things so clean?

2. Memory test for the last year

On the flipchart record as many events as the group can remember. Have a cribsheet from one of the newspapers to jog memories.

3. A 'word of time' quiz

(from *Language and Word Activities* page 3)

The answers are all related to time. Ask the group to write down a word that fits each definition.

1. An age...era
2. A period of royal rule...reign
3. A youth aged between 13 and 19...teenager
4. Happening every year...annual
5. Mensal (this is a difficult question)...monthly
6. Psalms sung in the evening...vespers
7. One hundred years...century
8. Animal active in daytime...diurnal
9. Animal active at nighttime...nocturnal
10. Equal length day and night...equinox
11. Two weeks...fortnight
12. A special day...red-letter-day
13. Before its due time...premature
14. One thousand years...millennium
15. Evenings...eventide
16. After dinner (maybe walk or drink)...post-prandial
17. The month named after the god Mars...March
18. Sixty seconds...a minute
19. The witching hour...midnight
20. When the mice ran down...one o'clock

4. Calendar quiz

Ask the group in general.

1. What are the four seasons?...winter, spring, summer, autumn
2. How many months begin with a 'J'?...January, June, July
3. How many months end in '-BER'?...September, October, November, December
4. How many months have four letters?...June, July
5. How many months have six letters?...August
6. Which month has the least number of days?...February
7. Is April the third or fourth month?...the fourth
8. If Luke is born in January, how old is he in July?...six months
9. If Emma is six months old on 1 July, when was she born?...1 January
10. In which month is the shortest day?...December
11. In which month is Bonfire Night?...November

5. See how many words can be found in: NEW YEAR RESOLUTION.

6. Watch the film *Calendar Girls* – or, if the film is not available, see how many words can be made from the title.

Activity Evaluation Sheet

Date .... Activity theme...

Staff members
Did the group enjoy the activities?
Which activity was enjoyed most?
Which activity enjoyed least?
Did anyone not join in? Why not?
Did the staff enjoy the theme?
Any suggestions to improve the activities?